IAP
Textbook of
DOWN SYNDROME

IAP
Textbook of
DOWN SYNDROME

Editor-in-Chief

Shaji Thomas John
MD DCH DTM&H PGDAP FIAMS FIAP (Hon) FNDP
Chief of Pediatrics and Neonatology
Baby Memorial Hospital
Kozhikode, Kerala, India

Chief Academic Editor

Gayathri K
MD DNB (Ped) MNAMS
Consultant and In-Charge
Down Syndrome Clinic
Department of Pediatrics
Baby Memorial Hospital
Kozhikode, Kerala, India

Academic Editors

Menon PSN
MD MNAMS
Former Sub-Dean
Professor of Pediatrics
Consultant-in-Charge
(Pediatric Endocrinology and Genetics)
All India Institute of Medical Sciences
New Delhi, India

Sankar VH
MD DNB MNAMS (Ped)
FIAP DM (Medical Genetics)
Professor
Department of Medical Genetics
Government Medical College
Thiruvananthapuram, Kerala, India

Krishnakumar P
MD (Psychiatry) DCH DNB (Ped)
Former Director,
Institute of Mental Health and
Neurosciences
Kozhikode, Kerala, India

Krishna Kumar R
MD DM FAHA
Clinical Professor and Head
Division of Pediatric Cardiology
Amrita Institute of Medical Sciences
Kochi, Kerala, India

Forewords

**GV Basavaraja, Vasant M Khalatkar, Upendra S Kinjawadekar,
Yogesh N Parikh, Remesh Kumar R**

JAYPEE

JAYPEE BROTHERS MEDICAL PUBLISHERS
The Health Sciences Publisher
New Delhi | London

Jaypee Brothers Medical Publishers (P) Ltd.

Headquarters
EMCA House, 23/23-B
Ansari Road, Daryaganj
New Delhi 110 002, India
Landline: +91-11-23272143, +91-11-23272703
+91-11-23282021, +91-11-23245672
e-mail: jaypee@jaypeebrothers.com

Corporate Office
4838/24, Ansari Road, Daryaganj
New Delhi 110 002, India
Phone: +91-11-43574357
Fax: +91-11-43574314
e-mail: jaypee@jaypeebrothers.com

Overseas Office
JP Medical Ltd.
83, Victoria Street, London
SW1H 0HW (UK)
Phone: +44-20 3170 8910
e-mail: info@jpmedpub.com

EU GPSR Authorised Representative
Logos Europe, 9 rue Nicolas Poussin
17000, La Rochelle, France
Phone: +33 (0) 6 67 93 73 78
e-mail: contact@logoseurope.eu

Website: www.jaypeebrothers.com
Website: www.jaypeedigital.com

Inquiries for bulk sales may be solicited at: jaypee@jaypeebrothers.com

IAP Textbook of Down Syndrome

First Edition: **2026**

ISBN: 978-93-6616-400-7

Printed at: Sterling Graphics Pvt. Ltd. India

Dedicated to

My daughter Tina, who made me commit myself to the welfare of children with Down syndrome, and to all the little angels with Down syndrome and their parents who stimulated me to surge ahead in my journey to make life better for persons with this condition.

Contributors

Abhay Mani Martin
MD DVD DNB
Senior Consultant and Head
Department of Dermatology
Baby Memorial Hospital
Kozhikode, Kerala, India

Anurag Gupta
MDS PGDMLS
Consultant Orthodontist
Certified Invisalign Provider
and Implantologist
Maximus Dental Center
New Delhi, India
Co-Founder, Smile Special Foundation

Balu Vaidyanathan
MD DM FACC
Professor, Pediatric Cardiology
Head
Division of Fetal Cardiology
Amrita Institute of Medical Sciences
Kochi, Kerala, India

Easwar T Ramani
MBBS DNB (Orth) MNAMS Fellowship in Pediatric Orthopaedics, Fellowship in Paediatric Deformity Correction and Scoliosis
Senior Consultant
Pediatric Orthopedics
Baby Memorial Hospital
Kozhikode, Kerala, India

Fayeda TK
MASLP MA (Psychology)
Assistant Professor
Department of Audiology and Speech Language Pathology
BM College of Allied Medical Sciences
Kozhikode, Kerala, India

Gayathri K
MD DNB (Ped) MNAMS
Consultant and In-Charge
Down Syndrome Clinic
Department of Pediatrics
Baby Memorial Hospital
Kozhikode, Kerala, India

Jayaraj MK
MA MSc MPhil PhD
Director
ULCCS Foundation
Kozhikode, Kerala, India

Krishna Kumar R MD DM FAHA
Clinical Professor and Head
Division of Pediatric Cardiology
Amrita Institute of Medical Sciences
Kochi, Kerala, India

Krishnakumar P
MD (Psychiatry) DCH DNB (Ped)
Former Director
Institute of Mental Health
and Neurosciences
Kozhikode, Kerala, India

KS Mohan
MD (Psychiatry) DPM (NIMHANS)
Former Professor and Head
Department of Psychiatry
Government Medical College
Kozhikode, Kerala, India

Leila Mohan
MS (Ophthalmology) DO Fellowship in Anterior Segment Microsurgery & Phacosurgery
Head
Department of Pediatric
Ophthalmology
Director Comtrust Academy
Comtrust Eye Hospital
Kozhikode, Kerala, India

Manoj MP
MS (ENT)
Consultant Otolaryngologist and
Cochlear Implant Surgeon
Unit of Head and Neck Surgery
MESIARC ENT Hospital
Kozhikode, Kerala, India

Menon PSN
MD MNAMS
Former Sub-Dean
Professor of Pediatrics
Consultant-in-Charge
(Pediatric Endocrinology and Genetics)
All India Institute of Medical Sciences
New Delhi, India

Mohandas Nair Karippoth
MD (Ped)
Professor
Department of Pediatrics
Government Medical College
Kozhikode, Kerala, India

Muhlisa V
MD (Physical Medicine & Rehabilitation)
Consultant Physiatrist
Department of Physical Medicine
and Rehabilitation
Baby Memorial Hospital
Kozhikode, Kerala, India

Neerja Gupta
MD DM (Medical Genetics)
Additional Professor
Division of Genetics
Department of Pediatrics
All India Institute of Medical Sciences
New Delhi, India

Neethu Koroth
BASLP Certified Level 2 OPT Practitioner
Diploma in Child Psychology
Consultant Audiologist and
Speech Language Pathologist
Baby Memorial Hospital
Kozhikode, Kerala, India

Nidhi Gupta
MDS
Consultant Endodontist and Cosmetic
Surgeon Special Care Dentist
Maximus Dental Center
New Delhi, India
Co-Founder, Smile Special Foundation

Rasitha Harish
MASLP
Head
Department of Audiology and Speech Language Pathology
Baby Memorial Hospital
Kozhikode, Kerala, India

Riya Lukose
DCH DNB (Ped) MRCPCH IAP Fellowship in Developmental and Behavioural Pediatrics
Associate Professor
Department of Pediatrics
Amala Institute of Medical Sciences
Thrissur, Kerala, India

Riyaz Arakkal
MD (Ped) DCH DNB DM (GE) FRCP
Professor and Head
Department of Pediatrics
KMCT Medical College
Kozhikode, Kerala, India

Sankar VH
MD DNB MNAMS (Ped) FIAP
DM (Medical Genetics)
Professor
Department of Medical Genetics
Government Medical College
Thiruvananthapuram, Kerala, India

Selvamanojkumar S
MD DM (Medical Genetics)
Division of Genetics
Department of Pediatrics
All India Institute of Medical Sciences
New Delhi, India

Shaji Thomas John
MD DCH DTM&H PGDAP FIAMS
FIAP (Hon) FNDP
Chief of Pediatrics and Neonatology
Baby Memorial Hospital
Kozhikode, Kerala, India

Sharada Mohan
MA MPhil PhD
Clinical Psychologist
Thondayad, Mavoor Road
Kozhikode, Kerala, India

Sheela Nampoothiri
DCH DNB (Ped) MSc Medical Genetics (Glasgow)
Clinical Professor and Head
Department of Pediatric Genetics
Amrita Institute of Medical Sciences
Kochi, Kerala, India

Sonia Karapurkar
MD DNB (Ped) FCPC (Ped Cardiology)
Fellow Fetal Cardiology (AIMS, Kochi)
Junior Consultant
Department of Pediatric and Fetal Cardiology
Jupiter Hospital
Thane, Maharashtra, India

Sreerenthu S Viswan
BASLP MSc (Speech)
Assistant Professor
Department of Audiology and Speech Language Pathology
BM College of Allied Medical Sciences
Kozhikode, Kerala, India

Vijayakumar M
MD DNB (Ped) FRCP
Professor and Head
Department of Pediatrics
Government Medical College
Kozhikode, Kerala, India

Foreword

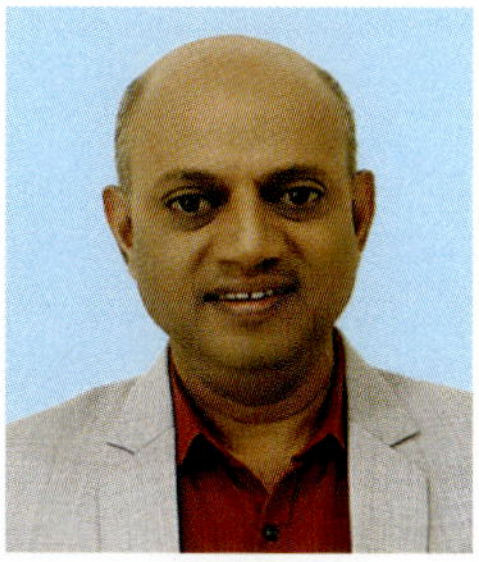

It is with great honor and anticipation that I write the foreword for this pioneering *IAP Textbook on Down syndrome*, a monumental contribution to the field of child health in India. This book addresses a vital yet often overlooked area of pediatric care, offering a comprehensive resource for medical professionals dedicated to improving the lives of individuals with Down syndrome.

Down syndrome, or trisomy 21, is a condition with profound medical, developmental, and social implications. While its diagnosis is straightforward, the true challenge lies in providing holistic care that addresses the complex needs of these individuals and their families. In India, where awareness and structured support systems are still evolving, this book comes as a much-needed guide to bridge the gap between diagnosis and meaningful, lifelong intervention.

The *IAP Textbook of Down Syndrome* is unique in its approach, blending clinical management with early intervention strategies, habilitation, and an emphasis on family-centered care. Its chapters, authored by a distinguished panel of 29 experts from across the country, delve into not only the medical but also the legal, educational, and social dimensions of care. This multifaceted perspective ensures that the book serves as a practical and empathetic guide for doctors, general pediatricians, and medical students alike.

As the first comprehensive reference textbook on Down syndrome from a developing country, this work holds immense significance. It highlights India's potential to contribute meaningful scholarship in the global medical community while addressing the unique challenges faced by families and practitioners in resource-limited settings.

I commend Dr Shaji Thomas John (Editor-in-Chief); Dr Gayathri K (Chief Academic Editor); and all the other eminent editors Drs PSN Menon, Sankar VH, Krishnakumar P, and Krishna Kumar R and the contributing authors for their tireless dedication to this project. Dr Shaji Thomas John's decades of experience in working with children with Down syndrome through the Down Syndrome Trust (DoST) form the cornerstone of this book's practical and compassionate insights.

This textbook is more than a resource—it is a testament to the power of collaboration, expertise, and unwavering commitment to creating a better world for individuals with Down syndrome. I am confident that it will inspire, educate, and empower its readers to bring about meaningful change in their practice and in the lives of countless families.

With my best wishes,

GV Basavaraja
Professor of Pediatrics
Indira Gandhi Institute of Child Health
Bengaluru, Karnataka, India
IAP National President, 2024

Foreword

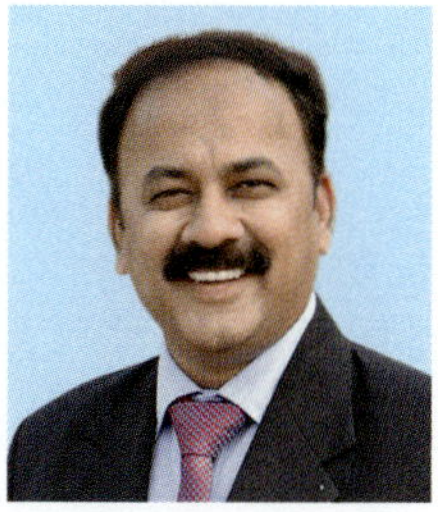

It is with immense pride and privilege that I present the *IAP Textbook of Down Syndrome*, a comprehensive guide designed to enrich the knowledge and skills of healthcare providers, educators, caregivers, and all those who play a pivotal role in supporting individuals with Down syndrome. This meticulously crafted textbook synthesizes years of rigorous research, clinical acumen, and lived experiences, offering a multidimensional understanding of Down syndrome.

Down syndrome, one of the most prevalent genetic conditions worldwide, occurs in approximately 1 in 700 live births and is characterized by an extra copy of chromosome 21. This genetic variation results in a spectrum of cognitive, physical, and developmental characteristics. However, it is imperative to recognize the unique individuality of every person with Down syndrome, as they demonstrate a wide range of abilities and potential. In this spirit, this textbook adopts a holistic approach, addressing not only medical and developmental aspects but also emphasizing psychological, social, and educational dimensions.

The opening chapters delve into the genetic and molecular mechanisms underlying Down syndrome, equipping healthcare professionals with a thorough understanding of its etiology and implications. Subsequent sections offer in-depth exploration of clinical manifestations, including frequently encountered challenges such as congenital heart defects, thyroid dysfunction, hearing impairments, and sensory processing issues. These chapters underscore the critical importance of early diagnosis, multidisciplinary management, and comprehensive care strategies.

A distinctive strength of the book lies in its focus on the social and educational contexts of life with Down syndrome. Contributions from leading experts in developmental psychology and education illuminate pathways for children with Down syndrome to thrive in diverse learning environments. This includes advocating for inclusive education, individualized interventions, and fostering robust family support systems. The emphasis on nurturing individual strengths and potential serves as a guiding principle throughout the book.

Additionally, this textbook addresses the key transitions that individuals with Down syndrome experience across their lifespan—from early childhood to adolescence and adulthood. With a focus on person-centered care, it offers practical strategies to empower individuals with Down syndrome to lead lives filled with purpose and dignity while promoting active family engagement and community participation.

This book is not just an academic resource but also a beacon for creating a more inclusive, empathetic, and supportive society. The collective expertise of its contributors reflects the progress we have made in understanding Down syndrome while reinforcing the importance of equity, respect, and opportunity for all.

I firmly believe that the book will serve as an indispensable resource for improving the quality of care and life for individuals with Down syndrome and for guiding the families and professionals who support them. May this textbook inspire a shared commitment to fostering a world where every individual, regardless of ability, can realize their fullest potential.

Vasant M Khalatkar
Consultant Pediatrician
Colours Hospital, Nagpur, Maharashtra, India
IAP National President, 2025

Foreword

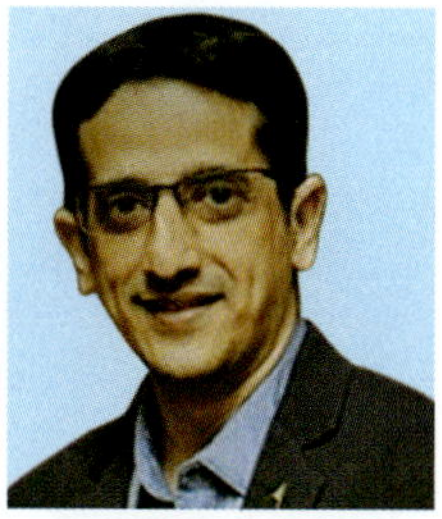

The English physician John Langdon Down was among the first to describe the disorder, now called Down syndrome (DS), about 150 years ago. Now we know that DS is the most common live-compatible human chromosomal abnormality, occurring in 1 in 700–800 newborns. The landmark discovery of human trisomy 21 as the chromosomal basis for DS has also positioned this disorder as the most complex human genetic disease compatible with postnatal survival. Individuals with DS often face unique developmental, cognitive, and behavioral challenges at various stages of development across the lifespan. The publication of the *IAP Textbook of Down Syndrome*, edited by Drs Shaji Thomas John, Gayathri K, PSN Menon, Sankar VH, Krishnakumar P, and Krishna Kumar R, is welcome news, which will provide the latest information on medically important areas associated with DS, including the prevalence; genetics; antenatal diagnosis; cardiac, skeletal, and dental abnormalities; and biochemical, respiratory, gastrointestinal, psychological, endocrine changes, etc.

Understanding the neuropsychological phenotype across the lifespan and the associated clinical, educational, and treatment needs is particularly important because of recent increases in life expectancy in DS due to improved health care, advocacy, services, and societal changes.

As primary care pediatricians, it is our responsibility to guide parents of children with DS not only about the medical problems but also on counseling, schooling, vocational issues, support groups, various insurance schemes and at the same time, caution them about controversial trends in the management. I am happy to say that his book has ensured to include each of these areas in great detail.

The authors and editors should be applauded for completing the book not before sharing some success stories which will definitely help the families and caretakers of children with DS while facing challenges thrown at them with a positive mindset.

I strongly recommend this book for every pediatrician, family physician, and obstetrician as well as for all those caring for children with DS.

Each child is unique and deserves the best!

Upendra S Kinjawadekar
Kamalesh Mother and Child Hospital and
Apollo Hospitals, Navi Mumbai, Maharashtra, India
National President, 2023
Indian Academy of Pediatrics

Foreword

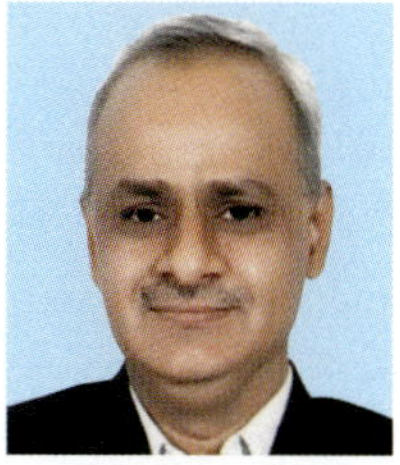

It is with great honor and privilege that I introduce the *IAP Textbook of Down Syndrome*, a comprehensive and invaluable resource dedicated to the understanding, management, and support of individuals with Down syndrome. This textbook represents a significant milestone in the field of pediatric healthcare, offering a wealth of knowledge and insights from leading experts and practitioners.

The book covers a wide range of topics, including the genetic basis of Down syndrome, early diagnosis and intervention, medical and developmental challenges, educational strategies, and the psychosocial aspects of care. Each chapter is meticulously crafted to provide a holistic understanding of the condition, emphasizing the importance of a multidisciplinary approach in addressing the diverse needs of individuals with Down syndrome.

As we continue to advance our knowledge and understanding of Down syndrome, it is crucial to recognize the contributions of individuals with Down syndrome and their families, who inspire us with their strength, determination, and love. This textbook is a testament to the collaborative efforts of healthcare professionals, researchers, and advocates who are dedicated to improving the lives of those affected by Down syndrome.

I extend my heartfelt gratitude to the authors, editors, and contributors who have made this textbook possible. Their expertise, dedication, and passion are evident in every page, making this an essential resource for anyone involved in the care and support of individuals with Down syndrome.

It is my sincere hope that the book will serve as a beacon of knowledge, compassion, and hope, guiding us towards a future where individuals with Down syndrome can thrive and achieve their fullest potential.

Yogesh N Parikh
Associate Professor
Department of Pediatrics
Government Medical College
Surat, Gujarat, India
Secretary General, 2024 and 2025
Indian Academy of Pediatrics

Foreword

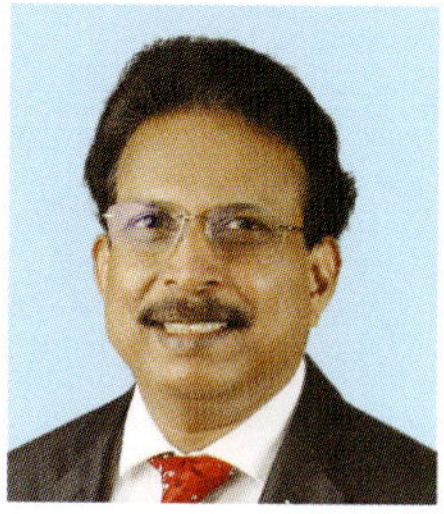

It is an honor and privilege to pen the foreword to this invaluable textbook on Down syndrome by Dr Shaji Thomas John, a luminary in the field of pediatrics and a steadfast advocate for children with Down syndrome and their families. As a renowned pediatrician and a guiding light for countless Down syndrome support groups, Dr John has dedicated his life to transforming both medical care and societal perspectives surrounding this condition.

This book is a testament to Dr Shaji John's profound expertise, compassion, and relentless commitment to enhancing the quality of life for children with Down syndrome. It serves as a comprehensive guide, bridging the gap between cutting-edge medical knowledge and practical, empathetic care. For pediatricians, this book offers a well-researched and practical framework for understanding the medical, developmental, and psychosocial needs of these children. For the general public, it demystifies the complexities of Down syndrome, fostering understanding, inclusion, and empowerment.

What sets this work apart is the unique ability of Dr Shaji Thomas John and his team of co-authors to balance scientific rigor with a heartfelt narrative. Drawing on decades of clinical experience and personal involvement with families, the authors present a nuanced exploration of the condition—highlighting not just the challenges but also the unique strengths and potential of individuals with Down syndrome.

In today's world where inclusivity and awareness are becoming cornerstones of healthcare and society, this book stands as a beacon of hope and education. Dr John's insights and guidance will undoubtedly inspire pediatricians to provide more holistic care and encourage families to embrace a journey of love, growth, and resilience.

This textbook is more than a resource; it is a movement—a call to action for a more compassionate and informed approach to Down syndrome. I am confident it will leave an indelible impact on its readers and contribute significantly to the ongoing efforts toward inclusivity and advocacy.

With great admiration and respect.

Remesh Kumar R
Director (Medical Services) and Senior Consultant (Pediatrics)
Apollo Adlux Hospital, Kochi
President, Indian Academy of Pediatrics 2022
Hon Secretary General, Indian Academy of Pediatrics, 2018 and 2019

Prologue

In the mid-1990s, an infant was brought to my outpatient room with acute respiratory infection. On examination, I found that the child also had Down syndrome phenotype with congenital heart disease. I was not sure whether the mother of the baby knew about this, and I was not knowledgeable nor trained to do proper counseling. So, I wrote a prescription for her respiratory problem and asked the mother to meet me after a week when the symptoms of cough and cold subsided.

"Doctor, does my child have a cardiac problem?"

"Yes." I was relieved to some extent because I did not have to break that news on follow-up.

"Doctor, does my child have Down syndrome?"

So, she knew about the condition as well and discussing about it would be easier for me.

I slowly said, "Yes."

As she was about to leave my room, she said, "Why are all the doctors so cruel?"

I was taken aback. Did I say or do anything that hurt her?

I have taken my baby to very many doctors including many in the neighboring states also. They just take one look at her and exclaim 'Oh! this baby has Down syndrome. Nothing can be done, don't waste your time running around.'

'This condition may be 1 in 800 for you, but it is 100% for me.'

And I remembered the status of my daughter Tina, who has Down syndrome.

That was when I realized that a lot had to be done for the benefit of the parents, the public, and the medical fraternity. As a first step, the Down Syndrome Trust (DoST) was formed in October 2000, and now more than 2,000 children with Down syndrome have benefitted from the venture.

And that infant is now a professional model and a calendar girl!

Shaji Thomas John

Acknowledgments

Writing some of the chapters and editing this book has been a meaningful journey, and I am deeply grateful to those who supported me along the way.

First of all, I wish to express my heartfelt gratitude to the Indian Academy of Pediatrics (IAP) for helping me to bring out this book which will be of immense benefit to all those interested in childcare.

I wish to acknowledge the inputs given by all the editors and for their unwavering support and encouragement. Our thanks go to the various authors who contributed to this book and shared with us their experiences in this field.

My sincere thanks go to Dr GV Basavaraja, the Immediate Past National President of the Indian Academy of Pediatrics (IAP), for the support given in bringing out this book and making it a reality. Thanks also go to Dr Yogesh N Parikh, Hony. Secretary General of IAP, for his involvement and guidance during the process of getting this book published. I wish to thank the National President, Dr Vasant M Khalatkar and the Past National President, Dr Upendra S Kinjawadekar (2023) for all the support given to us. I thank Dr Remesh Kumar R, the past National President, who kept me inspired and motivated in every stage of the process.

My thanks to Past IAP National President Dr MKC Nair, Past Chairperson Dr Jeeson C Unni, and Dr Kawaljit Singh Multani, Chairperson 2025 of IAP Chapter of Neurodevelopmental Pediatrics, for all the support given to me during the conception of the book.

I wish to thank M/s Jaypee Brothers Medical Publishers (P) Ltd, New Delhi, India for accepting to publish this book and for all the guidance given in shaping this book into what it is today.

I also wish to acknowledge the broader community of the special children with Down syndrome and their parents whose interactions and inputs helped spark the concepts and themes explored in this book.

I am indebted to Asia Pacific Down Syndrome Federation (APDSF) and the Down Syndrome Federation of India (DSFI) for emphasizing the need for such a book in the Asia Pacific region, which prompted me to take up the challenge to come out with such a book.

I am also thankful to Down Syndrome Trust (DoST) and the "DoST Support Group" whose belief in me kept me motivated to continue forward and taught me the practical lessons in management of these children from the parents' point of view.

I extend my heartfelt thanks to Dr KG Alexander and the management of Baby Memorial Hospital who provided me with a platform to cater to these children right from the year 2000 and to all my colleagues in the hospital who facilitated in the running of the Down Syndrome Clinic.

Last but not least, I thank my daughter Tina and my family who supported me and made this a reality.

This book is a testament to the collaborative spirit of everyone who touched it. I am forever grateful to all those who helped me and supported me.

Shaji Thomas John

Contents

SECTION 1: GENERAL CONSIDERATION

SECTION 2: SYSTEMIC MANIFESTATIONS

SECTION 1

General Consideration

CHAPTER 1

History of Trisomy 21

Shaji Thomas John

INTRODUCTION

Trisomy 21 or Down syndrome (DS) is a genetic disorder caused by the presence of all or part of a third copy of chromosome 21. The majority of mothers of babies with DS in developing countries are in the 20s, as pregnancy >35 years is comparatively less common in these countries. The management of DS has evolved from a purely medical model to a social and, now, a rights model. Regular and repeated counseling of parents is of utmost importance to ensure a sustained management program. Awareness and educational programs for the public at large are important to create an inclusive society in which these children can lead an independent life.

The history of DS is marked by significant advancements in medical science, shifts in societal attitudes, and ongoing efforts to improve the lives of individuals with the condition. From early descriptions by John Langdon Down to the discovery of its chromosomal basis by Jérôme Lejeune and the current emphasis on inclusion and advocacy, the understanding and support for individuals with DS have come a long way.

The stress on biopsychosocial strategy for the management of children with DS is reiterated, and the need for a medical, social, and rights model is recommended. Caregivers should be counseled and medical personnel sensitized and trained to provide appropriate management.

The history of DS involves the recognition and understanding of the condition over time, including its medical, social, and scientific aspects.

HISTORICAL ASPECTS

Ancient Times

Historical records suggest that individuals with characteristics of DS may have existed throughout human history. Some historians believe that artwork and literature from ancient civilizations, such as the Toltecs and the Greeks, depict people with DS, though these interpretations are speculative.

Middle Ages

Descriptions of individuals with physical characteristics similar to those seen in DS appear in some medieval writings, but the condition was not recognized as a distinct syndrome.

19th Century—Initial Recognition

The first description of DS was made by Jean-Etienne Dominique Esquirol in 1838 and later in 1844 by Édouard Séguin. But the condition was first described in a scientific manner by British physician John Langdon Hayden Down, who published an essay in 1866 titled "Observations on an Ethnic Classification of Idiots." He noted distinctive facial features and physical traits in some of his patients, who were intellectually disabled. Down referred to it as "Mongolian idiocy," a term based on his erroneous belief that it represented a regression to a more primitive human form. Down's work led to the term "Down syndrome" being used to describe the condition, although he did not understand its genetic basis.

20th Century—Chromosomal Basis and Nomenclature

The French geneticist Jérôme Jean Louis Marie Lejeune and his colleagues discovered in 1959 that DS is caused by the presence of an extra chromosome 21. This chromosomal anomaly thus came to be scientifically known as Trisomy 21, leading to the physical and intellectual characteristics associated with the condition. The condition became widely known as "Down syndrome," a term that is now preferred over various other terms. The older term "mongolism," which is considered outdated and offensive was abandoned in 1965. Morbus Langdon-Down, Morbus Down, Langdon Down disease, and congenital acromicria syndrome were the other names used earlier. Down's syndrome (with an 's) is used in England, Ireland, and some other English-speaking countries; whereas the term Down syndrome (without the 's) is the preferred term in the United States and Canada since 1974.

Late 20th Century to the Present Day

Advances in education and a greater emphasis on inclusion have allowed individuals with DS to participate more fully in mainstream education, employment, and community activities. There has been a shift from institutionalization to family-based care and support.

Advocacy organizations, such as Down Syndrome International (DSi), Global Down Syndrome Foundation, Asia Pacific Down Syndrome Federation (APDSF), Down Syndrome Federation of India (DSFI), and other international and local support groups have played crucial roles in raising awareness, promoting research, and supporting individuals with DS and their families.

Laws and policies, such as Baby Doe Law/Rules, brought in the United States as part of the 1988 Revision of the Child Abuse Prevention and Treatment Act (CAPTA), Indian Rights of Persons with Disabilities Act (PWD Act 1995), National Trust Act 1999, United Nations Convention on Rights of Persons with Disabilities (UN CRPD 2006), Rights of Persons with Disabilities Act (RPwD Act 2016) in India, and such others have provided legal protections and support for individuals with DS, ensuring their rights to education, employment, and community participation.

Research continues to improve understanding of DS, including studies on the genetic mechanisms, developmental challenges, and potential treatments. Scientists are exploring potential therapies and interventions that could mitigate some of the cognitive and health challenges associated with the condition.

MODERN UNDERSTANDING

Today, DS is understood as a genetic condition characterized by a range of physical and intellectual disabilities, with significant variability in severity among individuals. Modern medical care, early intervention, and supportive educational and social environments have greatly improved the outlook for individuals with DS, allowing them to lead fulfilling lives.

Advances in medical technology have led to the development of prenatal screening and diagnostic tests, such as amniocentesis and chorionic villus sampling (CVS), which can detect DS during pregnancy. Noninvasive prenatal testing (NIPT) has further improved the ability to screen for trisomy 21 using a blood sample from the mother. This has brought ethical and societal discussions about prenatal testing and the choices available to expectant parents.

Over the decades, medical care and therapeutic interventions for individuals with DS have significantly improved. Early neurodevelopmental interventions and specialized educational plans have enhanced the quality of life and developmental outcomes for those with the condition.

HOMO SAPIENS CHROMOSOME 21

Human chromosome 21 is the smallest human autosome, spanning approximately 48 million base pairs and representing about 1.5% of the total DNA in cells. The first published sequence of homo sapiens chromosome 21 (HSA21) annotated 225 genes on chromosome 21q. With increased knowledge of the elements of coding and noncoding genes and regulatory motifs, the number of gene structures recognized on HSA21 has increased considerably. The current version of GENCODE/ENSEMBL (GENCODE release 32) lists 233 protein-coding genes, 423 nonprotein-coding genes (69 small, 330 long, and 24 miscellaneous noncoding genes), and 188 pseudogenes. 48% of HSA21 has not been annotated, the vast majority of which contains repetitive elements (as is the case for all human chromosomes).

Chromosome 21 shares homology with a region on chromosome 16 in chimpanzees and other primates. Comparative genomics studies reveal that gene content and order are highly conserved, reflecting evolutionary stability. Phylogenetic studies help trace the evolutionary history of chromosome 21, shedding light on the divergence between humans and other primates and the evolutionary pressures that shaped its current structure.

STRUCTURAL VARIATIONS

Copy Number Variations

These are segments of DNA that are duplicated or deleted, leading to variations in gene dosage. Copy number variations (CNVs) on chromosome 21 can contribute to phenotypic diversity and susceptibility to diseases.

Partial trisomy 21 (PT21) is a rare genetic condition in which only a part of chromosome 21 is present in three copies instead of the usual two. Unlike full trisomy 21, where the entire chromosome 21 is duplicated (leading to DS), PT21 involves duplication of only a specific segment of the chromosome. This can occur due to an unbalanced translocation, where a segment of chromosome 21 is attached to another chromosome, or due to a duplication of a segment of chromosome 21 within the chromosome itself. The symptoms and characteristics of PT21 vary widely depending on the size and location of the duplicated segment. Some individuals with PT21 may exhibit features of DS, but typically in a milder form. Common features can include developmental delays, intellectual disabilities, and some of the physical characteristics associated with DS, but these may be less pronounced. PT21 is typically diagnosed through genetic testing, such as karyotype if the chromosomal duplication is large enough, or through chromosomal microarray analysis, which detects small duplications and deletions.

A highly restricted Down Syndrome Critical Region (HR-DSCR) of only 34 kb on distal 21q22.13 has also been identified as the minimal region whose duplication is shared by all subjects with DS and is absent in all non-DS subjects.

IMPORTANT GENES ON CHROMOSOME 21

- *Amyloid precursor protein (APP):* This gene is involved in the production of amyloid-beta peptides, which aggregate to form plaques found in the brains of Alzheimer disease patients.
- *Superoxide dismutase 1 (SOD1):* It encodes an enzyme that breaks down harmful superoxide radicals in cells. Mutations can lead to Amyotrophic lateral sclerosis (ALS).
- *Dual-specificity tyrosine-phosphorylation regulated kinase 1A (DYRK1A):* This gene plays a role in brain development and function.
- *Transmembrane protease, serine 2 (TMPRSS2):* This gene is associated with prostate cancer and has gained attention due to its role in SARS-CoV-2 infection. TMPRSS2 is a critical enzyme that facilitates the entry of SARS-CoV-2 into human cells by activating the viral spike protein. Its inhibition presents a promising therapeutic strategy for combating COVID-19. Ongoing research and clinical trials are focused on developing and evaluating TMPRSS2 inhibitors to provide effective treatments for COVID-19 and potentially other viral infections.

MEDICAL CONDITIONS ASSOCIATED WITH HOMO SAPIENS CHROMOSOME 21

- *Down syndrome:* The most well-known condition associated with chromosome 21 is Down syndrome (trisomy 21).
- *Alzheimer disease:* People with DS have a higher risk of developing Alzheimer disease, often at an earlier age. This is partly due to the overexpression of the *APP* gene.
- *Congenital heart defects:* A significant number of individuals with DS have congenital heart defects, necessitating specialized medical care.
- *Autoimmune disorders:* There is an increased prevalence of autoimmune disorders such as thyroid disease and celiac disease in individuals with DS.

GENETIC RESEARCH

Chromosome 21 has been extensively studied in genetic research due to its association with DS and other genetic conditions. It was one of the first chromosomes to be fully sequenced as part of the Human Genome Project. Ongoing research aims to understand the specific roles of genes on chromosome 21 and how their dysregulation leads to various health conditions. Techniques such as RNA sequencing provide insights into transcriptomic changes. Studies on DNA methylation and histone modifications on chromosome 21 help understand gene regulation and expression patterns, crucial for disease understanding and therapy development.

THERAPEUTIC INTERVENTIONS

This includes studies on gene therapy and targeted treatments. Significant efforts are directed toward understanding the mechanisms of trisomy 21 and developing interventions to mitigate the cognitive and physical challenges faced by individuals with DS. Research on chromosome 21 has implications for understanding various genetic disorders, cancer, and neurodegenerative diseases.

Emerging gene therapies aim to correct or mitigate the effects of gene dosage imbalances. For example, research is exploring ways to silence the extra copy of chromosome 21 in trisomy 21. Drugs targeting specific pathways affected by genes on chromosome 21 are being developed. For instance, inhibiting the overexpression of APP might delay the onset of Alzheimer in patients with Down.

Transgenic mice carrying human chromosome 21 segments are used to study gene function and disease mechanisms. These models help in testing potential therapies. Induced pluripotent stem cells (iPSCs), derived from patients with trisomy 21, are used to study cellular and developmental processes and screen for drugs.

LIFE EXPECTANCY OF PEOPLE WITH DOWN SYNDROME OVER THE YEARS

The life expectancy of individuals with DS has significantly improved over the years due to advances in medical care, early intervention, and societal changes. In the early 1900s, the life expectancy of individuals with DS was very low, often only reaching childhood. This was primarily due to a lack of medical understanding, inadequate healthcare, and societal norms that often led to institutionalization without proper care. By the mid-20th century also, life expectancy remained relatively low, with many individuals not surviving past their teenage years. Common causes of death included congenital heart defects, respiratory infections, and other medical complications that were not adequately treated.

During the 1980s, the life expectancy began to improve, reaching an average of about 25 years. The increase was largely due to better medical care, including corrective heart surgeries for congenital defects, antibiotics for infections, and a shift away from institutionalization toward family and community-based care. By the 1990s, life expectancy had further increased to approximately 35–40 years. This was a result of continued improvements in healthcare, early intervention programs, and the increasing availability of therapies and educational services. The development of vaccines and better management of respiratory infections also played a crucial role. As of the early 21st century, the average life expectancy for individuals with DS has risen to >60 years. Advances in cardiac care, the management of thyroid and other health conditions, improved support for mental health and well-being, and greater societal inclusion have all contributed to this increase.

SOCIETAL AND ETHICAL CONSIDERATIONS

Prenatal Screening and Diagnosis

Advances in noninvasive prenatal testing allow early detection of trisomy 21. Ethical considerations include informed consent, counseling, and potential impacts on decision-making.

Healthcare and Support

Improved understanding of chromosome 21-related conditions emphasizes the need for comprehensive healthcare, educational support, and social integration for affected individuals.

Public Awareness

Increasing awareness and understanding of conditions such as DS can reduce stigma and promote inclusion in society.

CONCLUSION

Down syndrome has been noted since ancient times, but it was only in the mid-19th century that the condition was recognized as a distinct entity. The chromosomal basis was identified only in the mid-20th century. Chromosome 21 has been extensively studied and research on gene therapy to correct or mitigate the effects of the extra chromosome is progressing with promising results in animal models. With better understanding of the condition, modern diagnostic methods, and therapeutic interventions, the life expectancy of persons with DS has risen, from death in the teenage period in the 1950s, to above 65 years now.

SUGGESTED READING

1. Antonarakis SE. Down syndrome and the complexity of genome dosage imbalance. Nat Rev Genet. 2017;18:147-63.
2. Down JLH. Observations on an Ethnic Classification of Idiots. In: London Hospital Reports. 1866;3:259-62.
3. Fraser BJ, Beldar S, Seitova A, Hutchinson A, Mannar D, Li Y, et al. Structure and activity of human TMPRSS2 protease implicated in SARS-CoV-2 activation. Nat Chem Biol. 2022;18:963-71.
4. Hattori M, Fujiyama A, Taylor TD, Watanabe H, Yada T, Park HS, et al. The DNA sequence of human chromosome 21. Nature. 2000;405:311-9.

5. Ko CJ, Hsu TW, Wu SR, Lan SW, Hsiao TF, Lin HY, et al. Inhibition of TMPRSS2 by HAI-2 reduces prostate cancer cell invasion and metastasis. Oncogene. 2020;39:5950-63.
6. LeJeune J, Gautier M, Turpin R. Study of somatic chromosomes from 9 mongoloid children [French]. C R Hebd Seances Acad Sci. 1959;248:1721-2.
7. Pelleri MC, Cicchini E, Locatelli C, Vitale L, Caracausi M, Piovesan A, et al. Systematic reanalysis of partial trisomy 21 cases with or without Down syndrome suggests a small region on 21q22.13 as critical to the phenotype. Hum Mol Genet. 2016;25(12):2525-38.
8. Pelleri MC, Locatelli C, Mattina T, Bonaglia MC, Piazza F, Magini P, et al. Partial trisomy 21 with or without highly restricted Down syndrome critical region (HR-DSCR): report of two new cases and reanalysis of the genotype-phenotype association. BMC Med Genomics. 2022;15:266.

CHAPTER 2

Chromosomal Basis of Trisomy 21 and Genetic Counseling

Sheela Nampoothiri

INTRODUCTION

Trisomy 21 is the most common genetic cause of mental handicap and is caused by three mechanisms. Even though the diagnosis of Down syndrome (DS) can be done by clinical evaluation, a karyotype analysis should be offered for all patients for identifying the type of DS.

1. *Nondisjunction type* ***(Fig. 1)****:* This is the most common type of DS, attributing to 90–95% of cases. They have 47 chromosomes with an extra chromosome 21 due to meiotic nondisjunction in the ovum in 95% of cases. The risk of nondisjunction increases with advancing maternal age **(Table 1)**.
2. *Translocation type* ***(Figs. 2 and 3)****:* The extra chromosome 21 is attached to any of the acrocentric chromosomes 13, 14, 15, 21, or 22. This contributes to 4% of cases, and 14;21 translocation is the most common among them. All patients with translocation type of trisomy 21 have only 46 chromosomes as the second copy of chromosome 21 is attached to either of the acrocentric chromosomes.
3. *Mosaic type* ***(Fig. 4)****:* This is the rarest type (1%). They have one cell line with 47 chromosomes with an additional chromosome 21 and a second normal cell line with 46 chromosomes. The most common mechanism for mosaicism is post zygotic nondisjunction where the zygote had normal chromosome complement and nondisjunction happens afterwards and this leads to a cell line with 47 chromosomes and another cell line with 46 chromosomes. When a probable mosaic type of DS is being evaluated, 100 metaphases should be analyzed for identifying a low-level mosaicism.

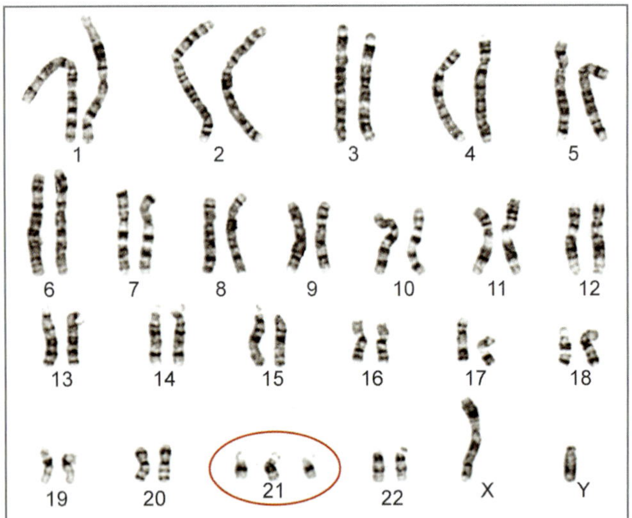

Fig. 1: Nondisjunction type of Down syndrome; 47,XY,+21.

TABLE 1: Risk of trisomy 21 with advanced maternal age.

20 years	1/1,500
25 years	1/1,350
30 years	1/900
35 years	1/380
41 years	1/85
45 years	1/28

MECHANISM OF NONDISJUNCTION IN DOWN SYNDROME

The process of gametogenesis is different in females and males. In females, primordial germ cells undergo 20–30 mitotic divisions and this occurs during the first 3 months of intrauterine life. Once the embryogenesis is completed by 3 months of intrauterine life, the oogonia begin to mature into primary oocyte which start to undergo meiosis I. At birth all primary oocytes would have entered into a phase of maturation arrest named as "dictyotene". Primary oocytes remain suspended until meiosis is completed at the time of ovulation when a single secondary oocyte is formed. Meiosis II then commences during which fertilization can occur. A very long interval between onset of meiosis in the fetal life and eventual completion

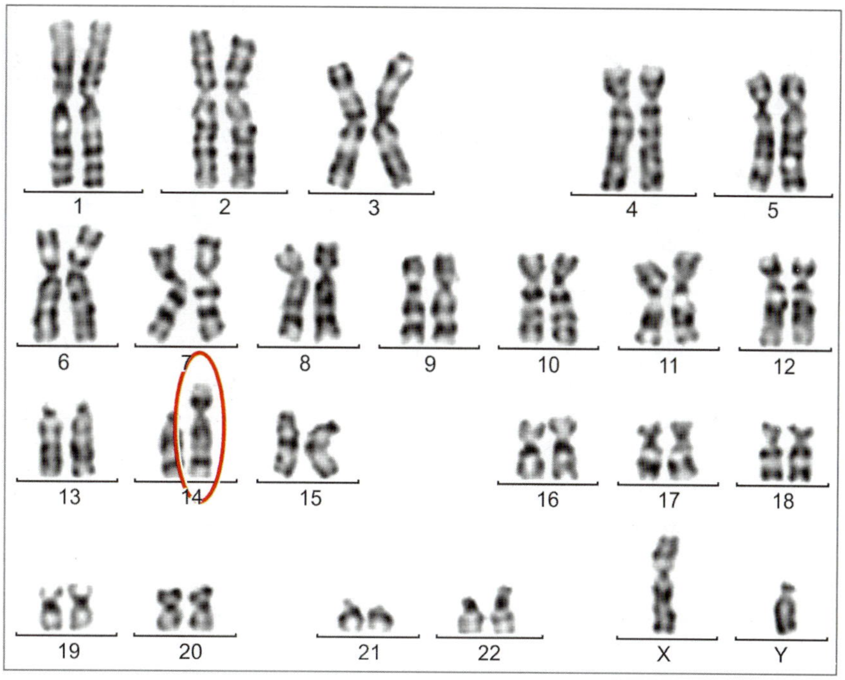

Fig. 2: Translocation type of Down syndrome. 46,XY,der(14;21)(q10;q10)+21.

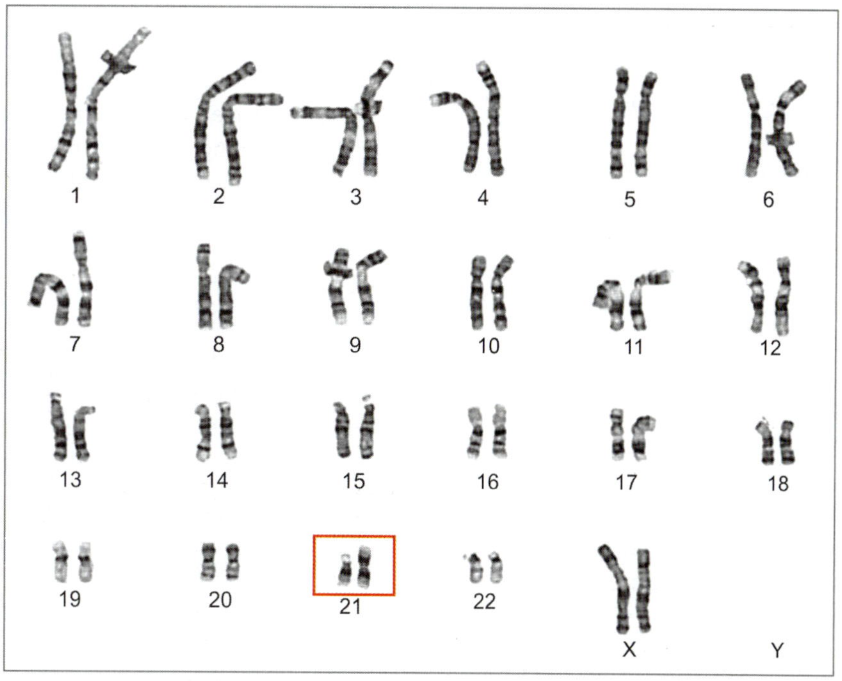

Fig. 3: Translocation type of Down syndrome. 46,XX,der(21;21)(q10;q10),+21.

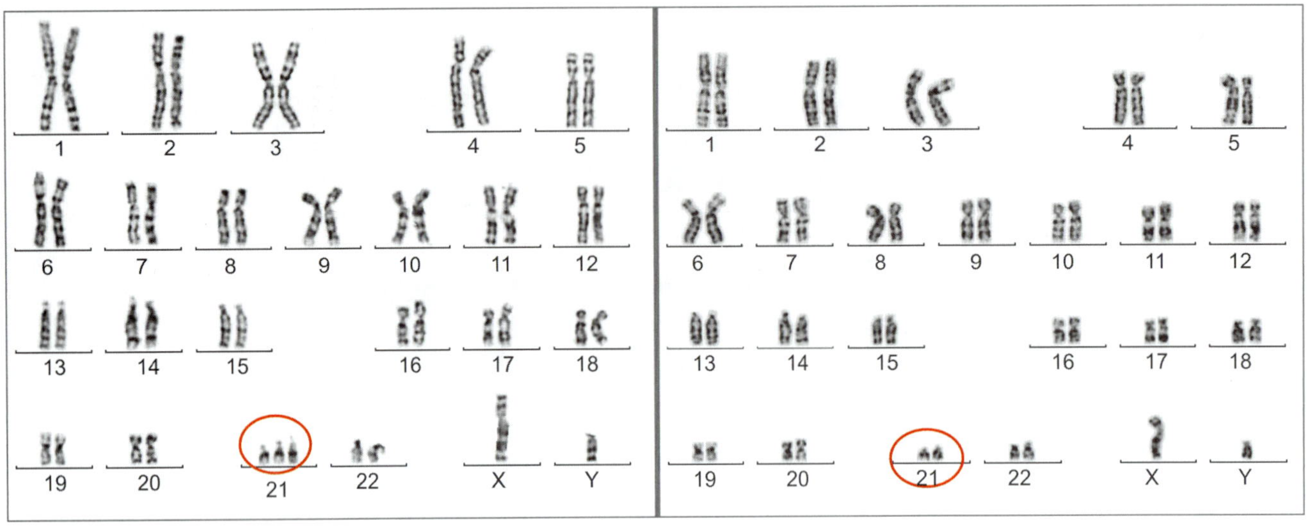

Fig. 4: Mosaic type of Down syndrome. 47,XY+21(70%)/46,XY (30%).

up to 40–50 years later leads to increased incidence of trisomies for the offsprings of elderly women. The wear and tear of primary oocyte during dictyotene phase probably damages the cell's spindle fiber function and repair mechanism which predisposes to nondisjunction. In contrast, spermatogenesis is a rapid process with average duration of 60–65 days. At puberty, spermatogenesis which has already undergone around 30 mitotic divisions matures as primary spermatocyte. They enter meiosis I and form secondary spermatocyte which in turn undergo second meiotic division to form spermatids and later to mature spermatozoa.

Trisomy 21 is usually caused by an error of maternal meiosis I. Rarely, it can be caused by meiosis II error as well when the sister chromatids fail to separate. In both these situations, the gamete receives two chromosome 21. When the gamete with two chromosome 21 fertilizes with a cell with single chromosome 21, it leads to the conception of a fetus with trisomy 21. The parental origin for meiotic errors leading to trisomy 21 is maternal (95%) and paternal (5%). Another cause for nondisjunction is absence of recombination in early prophase of meiosis I. The chiasmata that are formed following recombination is responsible for holding each pair of chromosomes until the separation occurs in late stage of prophase I. When the chiasmata formation is impaired, this would lead to the premature separation of the pair of chromosomes and they segregate randomly to daughter cells. In females, recombination occurs before birth but nondisjunction can happen any time between 15–50 years later. There is also a probable third factor which has been observed in Drosophila where there is some genetic control for nondisjunction. This must be the reason for recurrent nondisjunction occurring in few families.

ROBERTSONIAN TRANSLOCATION

This results from breakage of two acrocentric chromosomes (13, 14, 15, 21, and 22) at their centromeres with subsequent fusion of their long arms (q) and loss of short arms (p). The total chromosome number will be reduced to 45 for a carrier and they are phenotypically normal. The risk for being a Robertsonian translocation carrier is 1/1,000 among the general population and the most common translocation is between chromosomes 13 and 14 (13q14q).

For two-thirds of children with translocation type of DS, it would have occurred as a new event (de novo) and for the remaining one-third either of the parents would be a carrier. Once the parent has been identified as a carrier, every effort should be taken to trace other first-degree relatives to identify whether they are carriers for Robertsonian translocation so that they can be alerted regarding the probable risk to have a baby with DS in future pregnancy. This is called as "translocation chasing".

MOSAICISM

Chromosome mosaicism usually results from nondisjunction in early embryonic mitotic division, e.g., if nondisjunction happens during second mitotic division of the zygote, there will be three cell lines in a 4-cell zygote; two cell lines with 46 chromosome, one cell line with 47 chromosome (trisomy 21) and another cell line with 45 chromosome (monosomy 21). The cell line with monosomy 21 would not survive so that the resulting embryo will have around 33% mosaicism for trisomy 21.

COUNSELING

Recurrence risk for couples who have an affected child with trisomy 21 depends on the type of DS. The risk of DS increases with the advancement of maternal age and hence this parameter should also be considered while counseling the couple. A cross-sectional study conducted by Narayanan et al. on 418 children with DS from South India had shown that that 78% of children with DS were born to mothers <35 years. This highlights the need for universal first-trimester screening for all pregnant women.

For *nondisjunction type*, the recurrence risk is ~1%. Since the risk of Down syndrome increases with advancing maternal age, the couple should be offered the higher of the two risks. A parental karyotype is not indicated. Even though the risk of recurrence of nondisjunction trisomy 21 is estimated to be <1%, recurrence can occur very rarely. The two possible explanations suggested for the recurrence include low level mosaicism in either of the couple or a genetic predisposition to nondisjunction.

For *translocation type*, parental karyotyping should always be offered. If the parental karyotype is normal, the risk for the couple is extremely low as the translocation in the affected child is a "de novo" event (as a result of fresh mutation in the germ cell). If the father has a Robertsonian translocation involving chromosome 21 with any of these chromosomes (13, 14, 15, or 22), the recurrence risk is 1–3%, and if the mother is a translocation carrier **(Fig. 5)**, the risk is 10–15%. The exception is a 21;21 translocation carrier status in either of the parents, where the recurrence risk is 100% irrespective of the sex of the parent. Most of the 21;21 translocation type of DS are de novo.

For *mosaic type* of DS, the recurrence risk is negligible excluding the maternal age related risk and parental karyotype analysis is not warranted.

SPECIAL CASE SCENARIOS

- If a woman with nondisjunction type of trisomy 21 conceives, she has a 50% risk of having a child with DS.

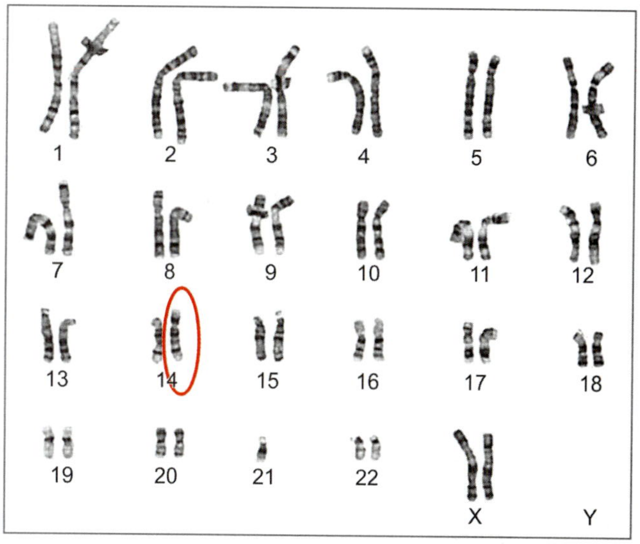

Fig. 5: Robertsonian translocation carrier, 45,XX,der(14;21)(q10;q10).

- A woman with mosaic type of DS has high risk for having an affected child with trisomy 21 and she should be offered amniocentesis in every pregnancy.
- If a couple with a normal karyotype has two pregnancies affected with nondisjunction type of trisomy 21, we should consider the possibility of gonadal mosaicism (either a few oocytes or sperms carrying two copies of chromosome 21 rather than a single copy) and they have around 10% risk to have an affected child in future pregnancy. Gonadal mosaicism cannot be confirmed by karyotype analysis from peripheral blood, and hence, the couple should be offered amniocentesis in subsequent pregnancies.
- Family history of DS in an uncle or aunt or sibling of the consultand (an individual who comes for genetic counseling): Obtain the karyotype of the affected individual, and if it is nondisjunction type, the risk is negligible. If it is a translocation type, karyotype of the consultand should be offered for ruling out the translocation carrier status. If the karyotype cannot be done for the affected person, the karyotype of a consultand should be done to rule out a small possibility of he/she being a translocation carrier.

CONCLUSION

Karyotype analysis should always be offered to all patients with Down syndrome to confirm the specific type, as this is essential for providing appropriate prenatal diagnostic options to the couple in future pregnancies.

SUGGESTED READING

1. Firth HV, Hurst JA. Oxford Desk Reference: Clinical Genetics and Genomics, 2nd edition. Oxford, UK: Oxford University Press; 2017; pp: 666-8.
2. Hook EB, Cross PK, Regal RR. The frequency of 47+21, 47,+18, and 47,+13 at the uppermost extremes of maternal ages: results on 56,094 fetuses studied prenatally and comparisons with data on livebirths. Hum Genet. 1984;68: 211-20.
3. Mueller RF, Young ID. (2001) Emery's Elements of Medical Genetics, 11th edition. Philadelphia: Elsevier Churchill Livingstone; 2001. pp. 42-52.
4. Nampoothiri S, Saadi AV, Girisha KM, Padmanabhan L, Yesodharan D, Thampi MV, et al. Recurrence of Trisomic Pregnancies in Four Families: A Cytogenetic and Molecular Study. J Fetal Med. 2019;6:81-7.
5. Narayanan DL, Yesodharan D, Kappanayil M, Kuthiroly S, Thampi MV, Hamza Z, et al. Cardiac spectrum, cytogenetic analysis and thyroid profile of 418 children with Down syndrome from South India: A cross-sectional study. Indian J Pediatr. 2014;81(6):547-51.

CHAPTER 3

Prenatal Diagnosis and Genetic Testing for Down Syndrome

Selvamanojkumar S, Neerja Gupta

INTRODUCTION

The diagnosis of Down syndrome (DS) is clinical; however, genetic testing using conventional cytogenetics is required. The mechanism of DS is maternal meiotic nondisjunction in 90% (paternal in 10%). The frequency of various types of chromosomal abnormality is listed in **Table 1**. In about a quarter, Robertsonian translocation is familial and has implications on recurrence risks. As patients with DS can have different cytogenetic abnormalities with different recurrence risk implications, it is important to have genetic testing for patients with DS.

METHODS FOR DETECTION OF DOWN SYNDROME

- Conventional cytogenetics for determining the origin of three copies of chromosome 21 (trisomy/translocation/mosaicism). It distinguishes between trisomy/translocation/mosaic DS **(Figs. 1A and B)** and has implications due to variable recurrence risks **(Table 1)**. Limitations of chromosomal analysis are a requirement of tissue culture and poor resolution.
- *Other diagnostic tests:* A rapid diagnosis of DS can also be made on interphase nuclei using quantitative fluorescent polymerase chain reaction (QF-PCR) **(Fig. 1C)** and fluorescence in situ hybridization (FISH).

Quantitative Fluorescence Polymerase Chain Reaction

The QF-PCR involves the amplification of specific polymorphic DNA markers (specific to chromosomes 13, 18, 21, X, and Y) across genomics after binding of fluorescently labeled primers that are specific to the region of interest. Measurement of the intensity of the fluorescent signal is measured by software and quantifies the copy number of each target chromosome. The procedure is automated and can be done from uncultured cells.

TABLE 1: Various etiologies of Down syndrome and its recurrence risks.

Type of chromosomal abnormality	*Frequency*	*Chromosomal abnormality*	*Recurrence risk*
Nondisjunction	95%	An extra copy of chromosome 21 (total number of chromosomes 47)	• Maternal age <35 years at previous trisomy 21, the revised risk is the age-related risk times 3.5 • Maternal age ≥35 at previous trisomy 21, the revised risk is the age-related risk times 1.7
Translocation	3–4%	An unbalanced structural chromosome rearrangement involving chromosome 21 (the most common translocation is between 14 and 21 chromosomes)	• If none of the parents is a carrier (de novo translocation in 75%), then the recurrence risk is <1% • Depends upon the type of translocation and parent of origin • If the mother is a carrier—10% • If Father is a carrier—1% • For translocation 21,21(either parent)—100%
Mosaic	1–2%	A mixture of cells containing both 46 and 47 chromosomes (due to an extra copy of chromosome 21)	Similar to that of nondisjunction trisomy 21

Source: Gardner RJM, Amor DJ. Gardner and Sutherland's Chromosome abnormalities and genetic counseling, 5th edition. New York: Oxford University Press; 2019.

A large number of samples can be handled at one time and results can be obtained within 24 hours which reduces the emotional stress of the couple. It has a sensitivity of 95% and a specificity of 99.9%. However, it can detect only aneuploidies of targeted chromosomes. **Figure 1C** depicts polymorphic markers for chromosome 21 showing three copies suggesting trisomy 21.

Fluorescence in Situ Hybridization

The FISH is one of the rapid detection targeted approaches for confirmation of aneuploidies. The fluorescently labeled region-specific probes of five common chromosomal aneuploidies (13, 18, 21, X, and Y) are hybridized on fetal cells, and fluorescent signals are obtained. Fluorescent signals obtained in a cell for each chromosome show the copy number of each chromosome. It can be done in uncultured cells and with interphase FISH trisomy 21 can be detected within 24–48 hours.

These tests are useful as there is no need for tissue culture, and the analysis is rapid. Interphase FISH also detects mosaicism.

Advanced maternal age is one of the most common risk factors for the occurrence of trisomy 21, though many babies with DS are born to women of young childbearing age. These children have developmental delay along with various comorbidities, especially cardiac anomalies which may be associated with high mortality. As per the American College of Obstetricians and Gynecologists (ACOG) and American College of Medical Genetics (ACMG), Society for Maternal-Fetal Medicine (SMFM) guidelines (2020), prenatal screening should be offered to all pregnant women regardless of maternal age. Prenatal screening

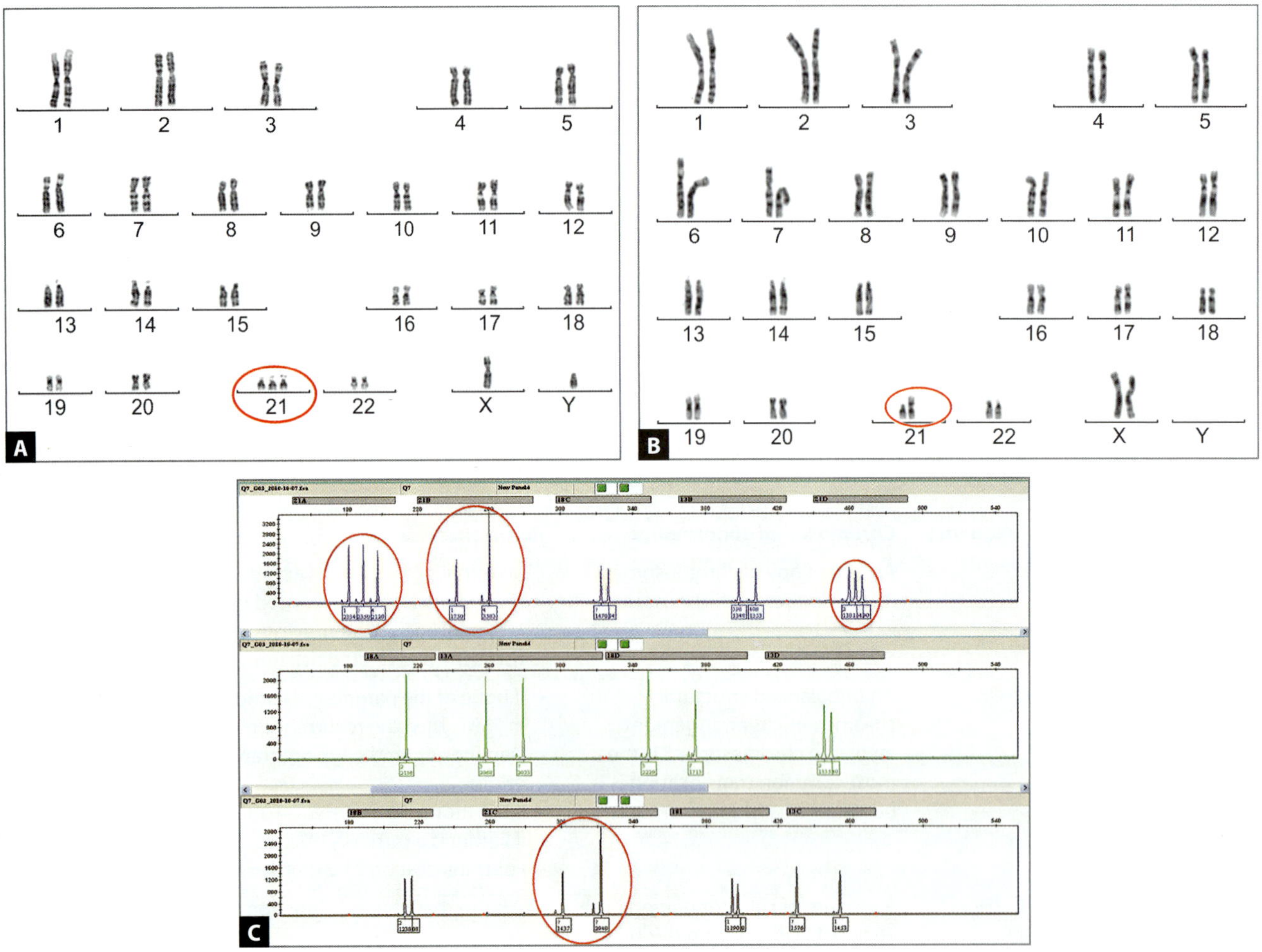

Figs. 1A to C: (A and B) Karyogram showing trisomy 21 and translocation (21:21) Down syndrome; (C) QF-PCR showing two markers in triallelic (1:1:1) ratio and two biallelic markers in 1:2 ratio for chromosome 21, suggesting trisomy 21. (QF-PCR: Quantitative fluorescence polymerase chain reaction).

Courtesy: (Fig. C) Dr Rashmi Shukla, Division of Genetics, Department of Pediatrics, AIIMS, New Delhi.

strategies for DS vary across different countries. The different screening tests are offered to pregnant women depending on the gestation, availability, and affordability of these tests.

PRENATAL SCREENING TESTS FOR DOWN SYNDROME

Pretest Counseling

This remains the prerequisite to any screening tests offered to pregnant women as each screening test has its limitations, different sensitivity, and specificity. The couple should be informed that these tests reveal only the risk of having a baby with DS or any other aneuploidy and must be confirmed by doing an invasive prenatal diagnosis if positive (high risk). They should be informed about screening test limitations, turnaround time, and the cost.

First-trimester Screening

First-trimester screening involves measurement of nuchal translucency (NT) at level I ultrasonography done at 11–14 weeks at a crown-rump length of 45 and 84 mm along with the measurement of free β-human chorionic gonadotrophic hormone (fβhCG) and pregnancy-associated plasma protein A (PAPP-A) levels in the maternal serum (combined test). The observed measurements are converted to multiples of the median (MoM) of unaffected pregnancies at the same gestation. Any values different from the defined normal MoM values confer a high risk of DS in that woman.

Measurement of NT should be done under standard ultrasonographic protocol during the stipulated period of gestation and crown-rump length. Increased NT is defined as a measurement above the 95th percentile for the normal range, according to the medians of the Fetal Medicine Foundation. Although increased NT is one of the risk factors for DS, other chromosomal aneuploidies, cardiac defects, fetal infections, anemia, and other monogenic causes should be considered while offering confirmatory testing. **Box 1** lists fetal ultrasonographic markers on the first-trimester scan.

BOX 1: Ultrasonographic markers on first-trimester scan.

- Increased nuchal translucency
- Hypoplastic/absent nasal bone
- Tricuspid regurgitation
- Reversal of ductus venosus flow
- Increased peak systolic velocity in the hepatic artery

First-trimester biochemical screening includes maternal serum measurement of fβhCG and PAPP-A (serum dual marker test). Typical patterns observed in DS pregnancies with twice high fβhCG and half the normal values for PAPP-A may not be seen in all. Confounding variables such as type of conception, maternal age, weight, ethnicity, and smoking status of women are considered while calculating the risk for various aneuploidies.

Screening by NT alone can detect only 80% of fetuses with trisomy 21 with a false positive rate of 5%. The combination of NT and biochemical screening improves the detection rate to 90%. The addition of other ultrasonographic markers along with serum screening can increase the sensitivity to 95% and reduce the false positivity rate to 3%. A risk value of 1:250 in combined screening confers a high risk for trisomy 21 whereas above 250 up to 1:1,000 confers an intermediate risk for trisomy 21 both of which should be followed by confirmatory testing.

In addition to DS, combined screening test also provides risk for trisomy 13, 18 and Turner syndrome.

Second-trimester Screening

Measurement of maternal serum α-fetoprotein (AFP), unconjugated estriol, and human β-chorionic gonadotropin is known as triple marker screening. Quadruple screening includes the addition of inhibin A to triple marker. It is performed between 15 and 22 weeks of gestation for trisomy 21, trisomy 18, and neural tube defect risk assessment. In pregnancies with DS, the hCG and inhibin levels were high and low estriol and AFP values. In trisomy 18, the levels of all three markers are decreased. With a 5% false positive rate, the sensitivity of triple screening is 65–70% and 70–75% for quadruple screening in singleton pregnancies whereas much lower to 50% in twin or more pregnancies.

The sensitivity and false predictive values of various tests are summarized in **Table 2**.

Second-trimester Ultrasonographic Markers

Various ultrasonographic markers were defined as soft markers for a chromosomal abnormality in the fetus during anomaly/level II ultrasonography. Those markers were renal pyelectasis, increased nuchal fold thickness, choroid plexus cyst, echogenic intracardiac foci, ventriculomegaly, echogenic bowel, short femur, intrauterine growth

TABLE 2: Sensitivity and false positive rates for various screening tests for Down syndrome.

Tests	*Sensitivity (%)*	*False-positive rate (%)*
MA + NT	75–80	5
MA + dual screening	60–70	5
MA + NT + dual screen (combined first-trimester screening)	85–95	5
Combined screening + additional USG markers (nasal bone or tricuspid flow or ductus venosus flow)	93–96	2.5
MA + quadruple screening	70–75	5
MA + triple screening	65–70	5
NIPS	99.9	1–2

Notes:
- Dual/double marker—free β-hCG (human chorionic gonadotropin) and PAPP-A (pregnancy-associated plasma protein-A)
- Triple marker—free β-hCG (human chorionic gonadotropin); AFP (alpha-fetoprotein), and uE3 (unconjugated estriol)
- Quadruple—triple + inhibin A

(MA: maternal age; NT: nuchal translucency; NIPS: noninvasive prenatal screening)

Source: Verma IC, Lall M, Dua Puri R. Down syndrome in India—diagnosis, screening, and prenatal diagnosis. Clin Lab Med. 2012;32(2):231-48.

retardation, and sandal gap. The presence of the above soft markers in absence/negative aneuploidy screening in the first trimester warrants further confirmatory testing for aneuploidies.

Noninvasive Cell-free DNA Testing from Maternal Blood

In early 2000, the discovery of cell-free DNA (cfDNA) testing of circulating fetal cells in maternal blood revolutionized prenatal testing for aneuploidies in pregnant women. cfDNA usually arises from the syncytiotrophoblast layer of the placenta and is released into the maternal circulation. The principle of the test lies in detecting a statistically significant increase in the relative dosage of chromosomal material in maternal cfDNA detected by next-generation sequencing or microarray hybridization to detect the presence of a trisomic cell line in the fetus. Noninvasive prenatal screening (NIPS) provides a sensitivity of 99.9% for the detection of trisomy 21 in singleton pregnancy.

A simple blood test (noninvasive), less turn-over time, and no risk to the fetus have made the initial choice of confirmation testing to rule out aneuploidies. In some developed countries, NIPS is being used as an initial screening test for aneuploidies, as it can be done as early as 10 weeks of gestation. Adequate fetal fraction (>4%) is required for interpretation of NIPS results. Maternal obesity, smoking, earlier gestation, and smaller placenta as in trisomy 13 and 18 are some of the causes of low fetal fraction. NIPS failure confers as one of the risk factors for a chromosomally abnormal fetus. Though it has high sensitivity, it remains a screening test and hence needs confirmation testing by invasive means if it turns out to be positive. The high cost of the test in the Indian scenario has been an deterrent deciding factor for couples.

In twin pregnancies, NIPS can be offered as an aneuploidy screening method in high-risk pregnancies after confirming zygosity. For diamniotic dichorionic (DADC) twins, separate fetal fractions and risk are obtained. A high false-positive rate can be due to a vanishing twin with aneuploidy in early pregnancy.

Post-test Counseling

Declaration of screening results should also be accompanied with post-test counseling especially if it turns out to be high risk. Information regarding definitive testing is given.

CONFIRMATORY PRENATAL TESTING FOR DOWN SYNDROME

Indications for prenatal diagnosis of DS are as follows:
- Any pregnant women with screening positive (either combined screening or NIPS)
- Any pregnant women with positive ultrasonographic soft markers
- Pregnant women with fetal malformations suggestive of DS such as atrioventricular septal defect, and double bubble sign.

All genetic testing requires pre- and post-test counseling. Pretest counseling for prenatal diagnosis helps the consultand to understand the overall outcome of the abnormality to enable them to decide about undergoing testing; the risk associated with the invasive testing, the cost, and the turnaround time.

Invasive testing requires fetal samples using chorionic villous sampling, amniocentesis, and fetal blood sampling depending upon the gestational age at presentation.

Chorionic villous sampling is the procedure of sampling chorionic villous tissue from the placenta after 11 weeks of gestation through transabdominal ultrasonography. Amniocentesis is the removal of amniotic fluid containing shredded fetal cells for testing between 16 and 20 weeks of gestation. Procedural-related risk of pregnancy loss is low, or negligible, especially by an experienced operator. Fetal cord blood sampling can be used as one of the sampling methods in late gestation testing.

Various methods are employed for conformational testing on fetal samples obtained depending on the availability and turnaround time of the tests.

Karyotyping

Karyotyping remains the gold standard testing for the detection of aneuploidies from cultured amniocytes or chorionic villous cells. It provides 100% sensitivity and specificity. However, it requires 10–14 days for cultured cells to grow and obtain results of stained smears. This prolonged turn-around time can create more anxiety for the couple. Hence rapid diagnostic tests such as QF-PCR/FISH as mentioned above can be employed in such situations.

In patients with additional nonspecific fetal malformations, a chromosomal microarray test should be done after ruling out common aneuploidies.

Counseling

Prenatal counseling does not end with testing and obtaining results. Breaking the bad news to the couple if it is abnormal and reassuring them if it is negative is a vital part of genetic counseling. If a fetus is affected with DS, parents should be counseled about the disorder, its course, and prognosis which helps in their further decision on pregnancy. Depending on the type of DS, recurrence risk should be explained to the couple **(Table 1)**.

CONCLUSION

Prenatal screening and detection of DS should be offered to all pregnant women due to mortality and comorbidity associated with the disease. As there are various tests available and risks associated with some of the procedures, proper pretest counseling is offered. The counseling about the choice of testing should be nondirective and should facilitate couple choice rather than direct advice.

SUGGESTED READING

1. American College of Obstetricians and Gynecologists Committee on Practice Bulletins—Obstetrics, Committee on Genetics, Society for Maternal-Fetal Medicine. Screening for fetal chromosomal abnormalities: ACOG Practice Bulletin, number 226. Obstetr Gynecol. 2020;136(4): e48-e69.
2. Benn P, Rebarber A. Noninvasive prenatal testing in the management of twin pregnancies. Prenat Diagn. 2021; 41(10):1233-40.
3. Gardner RJM, Sutherland GR. Chromosome Abnormalities and Genetic Counseling, 5th edition. New York: Oxford University Press; 2018.
4. Hui L, Ellis K, Mayen D, Pertile MD, Reimers R, Sun L, et al. A position statement from the International Society for Prenatal Diagnosis on the use of non-invasive prenatal testing for the detection of fetal chromosomal conditions in singleton pregnancies. Prenat Diagn. 2023;43(7):814-28.
5. International Society of Ultrasound in Obstetrics and Gynecology; Bilardo CM, Chaoui R, Hyett JA, Kagan KO, Karim JN, Papageorghiou AT, et al. ISUOG Practice Guidelines (updated): performance of 11–14-week ultrasound scan. Ultrasound Obstet Gynecol. 2023;61(1): 127-43.
6. Sahota DS, Leung TY, Chan LW, Law LW, Fung TY, Chen M, et al. Comparison of first-trimester contingent screening strategies for Down syndrome. Ultrasound Obstet Gynecol. 2010;35(3);286-91.
7. Salomon LJ, Sotiriadis A, Wulff CB, Odibo A, Akolekar R. Risk of miscarriage following amniocentesis or chorionic villus sampling: a systematic review of the literature and updated meta-analysis. Ultrasound Obstet Gynecol. 2019; 54(4):442-51.
8. Sheets KB, Crissman BG, Feist CD, Sell SL, Johnson LR, Donahue KC, et al. Practice guidelines for communicating a prenatal or postnatal diagnosis of Down syndrome: recommendations of the National Society of Genetic Counselors. J Genet Couns. 2011;20(5):432-41.
9. Verma IC, Lall M, Dua Puri R. Down syndrome in India—diagnosis, screening, and prenatal diagnosis. Clin Lab Med. 2012;32(2):231-48.

CHAPTER 4

Down Syndrome: Clinical Features

Mohandas Nair Karippoth

INTRODUCTION

The clinical diagnosis of Down syndrome (DS) is made "by Gestalt." It is not by looking for individual dysmorphic features, but by the overall appearance. But to have this Gestalt diagnosis, the clinician should be familiar with individual dysmorphic features also along with overall appearance. In a newborn with DS, the overall appearance is usually better appreciated when the baby cries.

Clinical diagnosis can be more difficult in the newborn period, and the clinician could be under stress as the implications of such a diagnosis are very large. So, it will be better to go by certain criteria, and Hall's criteria are a useful tool in such situations. This is composed of 10 components as depicted in **Table 1**. The approximate frequency observed for each component is also shown. Almost all babies with DS have at least four features and 89% have six or more.

CLINICAL FEATURES OF DOWN SYNDROME

Babies with DS have hypotonia. This is partly responsible for the gross motor developmental delay and dysarthria they manifest. As age advances, hypotonia decreases. Developmental delay is global, but receptive speech and social development are less affected. Moro reflex is poor in these neonates.

TABLE 1: Hall's criteria to diagnose Down syndrome clinically in newborn babies.

Neonatal sign	*Frequency (%)*
1. Hypotonia	80
2. Poor Moro reflex	85
3. Flat face	90
4. Upward slanted palpebral fissure	80
5. Small dysplastic ears	60
6. Joint hyperflexibility	80
7. Short neck and redundant skin	80
8. Short 5th digit with clinodactyly	60
9. Single transverse palmar creases	45
10. Pelvic dysplasia (radiological)	70

Craniofacial features: Children with DS have brachycephaly and a flat occiput. Even though brachycephaly is a visual impression, it can be objectively measured by calculating the cephalic index.

$$\text{Cephalic index (CI)} = \frac{\text{Biparietal diameter} \times 100}{\text{Occipitofrontal diameter}}$$

Normal is between 76 and 81. If CI is more than 81, it is brachycephaly, and if less than 76, dolichocephaly. They have a flat face, as their forehead and nose are almost in level with the rest of the face. The palpebral fissure slants upward. This is appreciated by drawing an imaginary line joining the two medial canthi. If the outer canthi are above this line, the palpebral fissures are considered as having up slant or mongoloid slant **(Fig. 1)**. If outer canthi are below this line, it is antimongoloid slant or down slant. The ears will appear apparently low set because the ear will be below the line joining the inner and outer canthi as there is mongoloid slant. To analyze whether the ear is low set or not, the line joining both inner canthi should be used and see how much of the ear is above this line. Usually, there will be a fold of skin which covers the medial canthus,

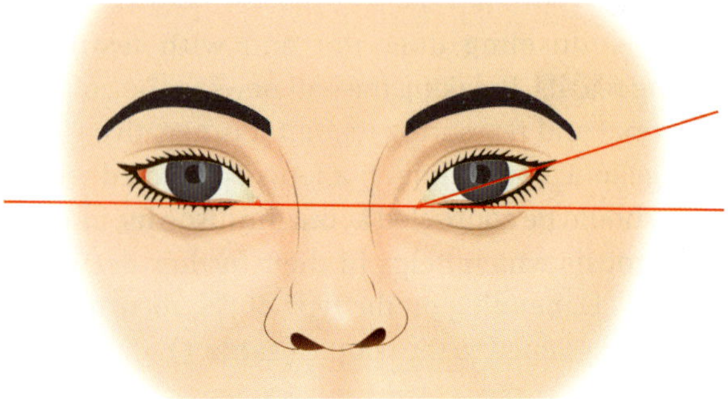

Fig.1: Upward slant of eye in Down syndrome (DS).

which is called epicanthic fold **(Fig. 2)**. The nasal bridge is often depressed, which, along with the epicanthic fold, gives an impression of hypertelorism. True hypertelorism can also occur, which is a situation where the eyes are placed wide apart. Here, the inner canthal distance, outer canthal distance, and interpupillary distance are all above the 95th centile **(Fig. 3)**. The iris of these children is described to have speckling, which is called Brushfield spots. This finding is less often seen in Indian children with dark irises. Other ocular findings include fine lens opacities, squint, nystagmus, keratoconus, and cataract.

Fontanelles are usually wide, and a third fontanelle may be palpable in newborns between the anterior and posterior fontanelles. The closure of the fontanelle is also delayed. The frontal sinus in these children is hypoplastic and so is the midface. The head circumference is less compared to normal, and in some children, the definition of microcephaly is fulfilled (3SD below the median value). The palate is short, the nose is small, with flattening of the nasal bridge. Mostly the tongue is of normal size, but it tends to protrude because of a small oral cavity. True macroglossia is also seen in some. The tongue often exhibits deep fissures. The corners of the mouth are turned down. The ears are small, rounded, and simple.

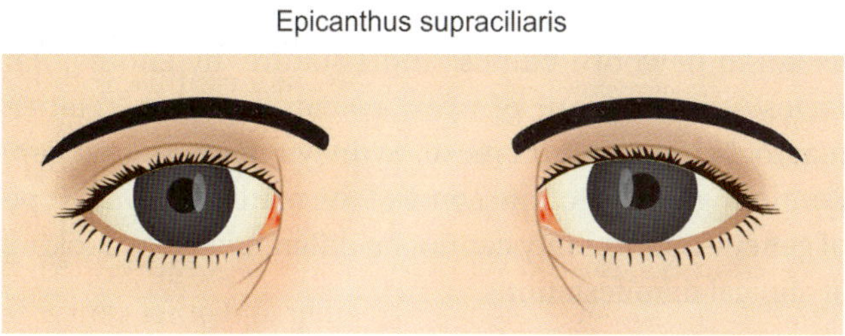

Fig. 2: Medial epicanthal fold in Down syndrome (DS).

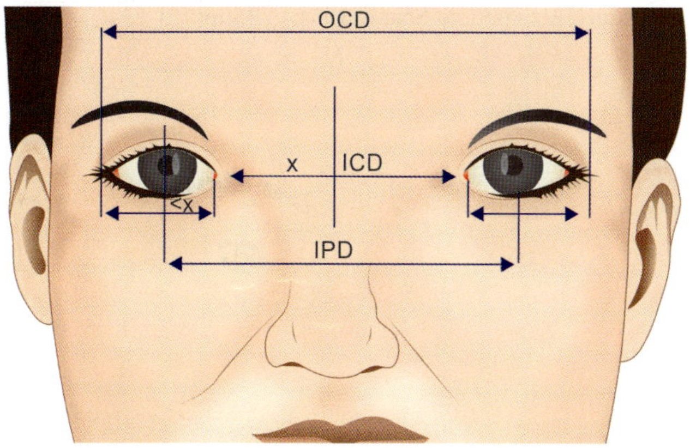

Fig. 3: Hypertelorism in Down syndrome (DS).

Hands and feet in DS were previously described as congenital acromicria because of the small size of hands and feet. This terminology is not in use now. The fingers are short. Long and slender fingers are highly unlikely in children with DS. The fifth digit is short and curved in with often a single interphalangeal crease because of hypoplasia of the middle phalanx. This dysmorphism is described as clinodactyly. Simian crease (single transverse palmar crease) is a finding much overstated in DS. Bilateral single palmar crease is seen in <50% of children with DS. One in 30 normal individuals has a unilateral simian crease and rarely bilateral also. Some children with DS have an extended proximal transverse crease which extends the entire width of the palm. This is Sydney crease **(Fig. 4)**.

The toes are also short. The gap between the big toe and the second toe is wide, described as a sandal gap. There is a deep groove between these two toes, which is named as Kennedy groove or Kennedy crease **(Fig. 5)**. The dermatoglyphic pattern is also distinct in DS. Hallucial tibial arch (in 72% of individuals) and a small distal loop (32%) in the big toe are observed in the sole. In hand, they have predominantly ulnar loops in fingers. The atd angle is obtuse as the palm is short and broad **(Fig. 6)**.

The scalp hair is often fine and straight. Curly hair is not very common. As they are prone to many autoimmune problems, premature graying of hair and patchy alopecia are not rare findings. Graying is mostly permanent, but hair can regain its color, and alopecia can recover, even though less frequent.

The most important skeletal change in DS is flaring of iliac wings, resembling elephant ears, also described as

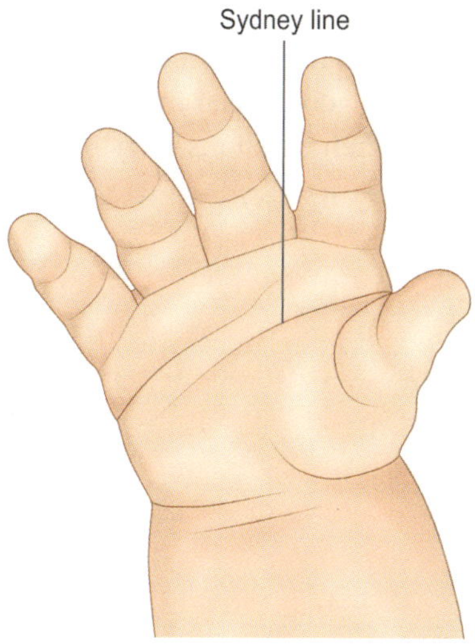

Fig. 4: Sydney line in Down syndrome (DS).

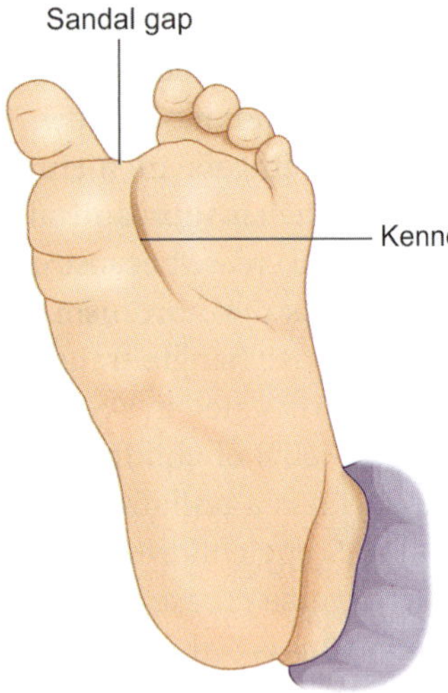

Fig. 5: Sandal gap and Kennedy groove in Down syndrome (DS).

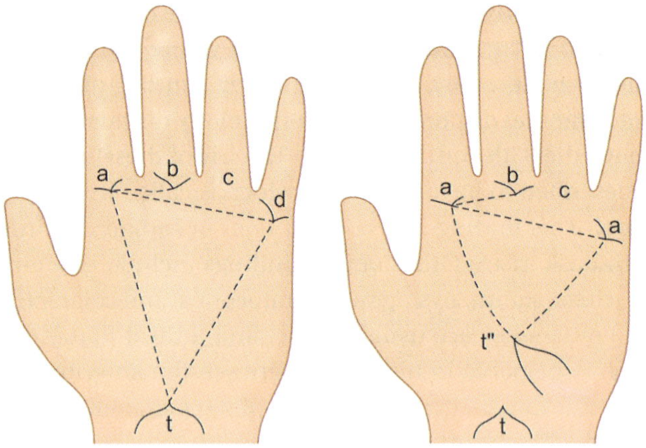

Fig. 6: Obtuse atd angle on the palms.

the Mickey Mouse sign. Brachymesophalangy of the fifth finger is another one. Almost one-third of children with DS have only 11 pairs of ribs. (In the general population, this variation is seen in 10% of individuals). Odontoid abnormalities are found in up to 16% of individuals with DS. Atlantoaxial instability is due to generalized congenital laxity of ligaments and odontoid abnormalities.

Palmoplantar hyperkeratosis is seen in almost half of the individuals. Xerosis and seborrheic dermatitis are other skin manifestations. Mongolian spots, which are normal findings in newborns, have got no association with DS (even though mongolism was the term previously used to denote Down syndrome).

Newborn babies with DS are frequently described as good babies. They are usually calm and composed. As children, they are happy, cheerful, good tempered, and humorous with good social interaction. They never hesitate to express their emotions even to strangers.

Short stature is seen in almost all children with DS. At birth, their length is 2–3 cm less than the average length of newborns. As they grow, the difference becomes more evident. Short stature is symmetric, with a normal upper segment to lower segment ratio for age.

CONCLUSION

Clinical diagnosis of DS is by gestalt. Hall's criteria is useful in newborn babies. Short stature, hypotonia, flat facies, upward slant of eyes, epicanthic folds, relative macroglossia, simian crease, Sydney crease, sandal gap, Kennedy groove etc., are some of the manifestations. Type of genetic abnormality cannot be differentiated by looking at clinical manifestations.

SUGGESTED READING

1. Hall B. Mongolism in newborns. A clinical and cytogenetic study. Acta pediatr Scand. 1964;154(Suppl):1-95.

CHAPTER 5

Development Aspects in Down Syndrome

Riya Lukose

INTRODUCTION

It is a well-known fact that individuals with Down syndrome (DS) have lower intelligence, but they are so much better when considering their socio emotional development. They have an IQ range from 10 to 70, with an average of 40, and they have predominant defects in executive function, which includes defects in attention, inhibition, organizational capacity, self-monitoring, etc. They also have problems in their, short-term, long-term, and procedural memory. Postmortem and magnetic resonance imaging (MRI) studies of the brain in individuals with DS have been shown to differ in the overall size of the brain when compared to age-matched controls. The major areas affected are the cerebral cortical hemispheres, cerebellum, and hippocampus. These brain structures, which are reduced in size in DS, are the ones responsible for executive function (frontal lobe, parietal lobe, and cerebellum) and memory (hippocampus). The differences in neuroanatomy have been demonstrated to be present not only from birth but from as early as 23 weeks in utero, and they have been shown to have a poor growth trajectory as the child grows; the volume loss of these parts of the brain being more prominent, especially after 3–5 months of life. In addition to these structural alterations, there is a reduction in the number of proliferating neural progenitor cells (NPCs) in the dentate gyrus, germinal matrix of the lateral ventricle, and third ventricle in fetuses diagnosed with DS (17–21 weeks gestation). Other neurodevelopmental processes such as dendrite arborization and synapse formation are also affected in DS. There are changes in myelination and changes in the astrocyte and glial population too.

In addition to all the neuroanatomic abnormalities, they have many comorbid conditions, which can also result in variation in their normal development. The parental care and nurture, family support, and definite early intervention are not to be forgotten in the development of children with DS. A foundational investigation was conducted by Ed Zigler and colleagues, who purported the "similar-sequence" and the "similar structure" hypotheses. The similar-sequence hypothesis suggested that children with intellectual disability (ID) follow a universal developmental progression, passing through stages sequentially similar to typically developing (*TD)* children. The similar structure hypothesis emphasized that cognitive structures would be similar among all children, and the way learning occurs would be similar in children with and without ID. These hypotheses were demonstrated in individuals with nonorganic causes of ID, but this similar-structure pattern was less frequently observed in individuals with organic causes of ID such as DS and William. It has been proved beyond doubt that DS infants do not follow the normal developmental trajectory. The development in each domain also differs in DS; many studies have been done to elaborate on the developmental milestones in DS.

MOTOR MILESTONES

The gross difference in the motor milestones when compared to TD individuals is due to the abnormal movement patterns, hypotonia, and hyperflexibility in this population. Delays in the emergence and disappearance of postural reflexes are also prevalent in this population. Dmitriev describes four different types of infants with DS based on muscle tone and motor functioning. Type 1 (15–25%) babies who have good muscle tone and attain milestones such as head control, bearing weight on feet with support, and lifting the torso on extended arms by 4 months. Types 2 and 3 (50–60%) babies show a variation between upper and lower body motor functioning. Type 2 infants have strong upper back, neck, shoulders, and arms but are unable to bear weight on their legs as other infants are able to do, whereas type 3 infants have strong legs and lower torso, but weaker upper torso, neck, head, shoulders, and arms. And the type 4 babies (15–25%) are weak all over, with flaccid arms and legs, and often have accompanying cardiovascular challenges. So, even if we can approximately predict the motor milestone in DS, there can be variations among this group itself, as we know no two individuals are similar. In addition to the motor delay, they also may have difficulty in motor planning, such as toddlers were seen to have difficulty in stringing beads. In a 1998 study by Jobling, 10- to 16-year-old children with DS had specific motor impairments, including difficulty with precise movements of limbs (e.g., stepping over a stick while on a balance beam) and fingers (e.g., pivoting thumb and index finger) as well as gross motor tasks such as sit-ups and push-ups. Tudella et al. reported that prior to the age of 7 months, infants with DS in their sample were delayed by 1 month relative to typical infants, but after 7 months, the degree of delay increased.

Kim et al. classified the motor and cognitive profiles of children with DS and put forward the timings of expected developmental milestones when compared to TD children. The average age at which the children with DS reached each motor milestone is noted in **Table 1**.

Children with DS were seen to be following the same sequence of motor development and generally take double the time to acquire developmental milestones when compared with other children. Moreover, it is clear from the above that there is a wide age range of estimates for motor milestones, there is a high degree of variability in skill acquisition, and, importantly, heterogeneity is present in developmental trajectories. Almost all children with DS showed a moderate degree of intellectual disability, and motor and cognitive development did not seem to correlate with one another.

TABLE 1: Difference between motor milestone achievement of children with Down syndrome (DS) and typical children (unit, month).

	Children with DS	*Typically developing children*	*Difference between the two groups*
Head control	6.1 ± 2.6	3.0	3.1
Turning	8.8 ± 3.1	5.0	3.8
Sit alone	11.9 ± 3.3	6.0	5.9
Creeping	13.9 ± 3.5	8.0	5.9
Crawling	18.1 ± 5.0	8.5	9.6
Cruising	22.3 ± 7.2	9.2	13.1
Independent walking	28.0 ± 8.3	12.1	15.9

Source: Kim HI, Kim SW, Kim J, Jeon HR, Jung DW. Motor and cognitive developmental profiles in children with down syndrome. Ann Rehabil Med. 2017;41(1):97-103.

LANGUAGE MILESTONES

Much research has been done regarding the cognitive and communication domains in DS. In fact, due to the increased numbers when compared to other intellectual disability syndromes such as Williams, Smith Magenis, Angelman, or Prader-Willi, DS has been the most researched. The various research can thus help us to find a foothold in either the prevention of severe disability or help us formulate the best ways for early intervention.

Studies that describe communication in DS have been done more during the first years of life. The DS language phenotype includes predominant impairments in expressive language relative to receptive language, with very poor vocabulary size relative to mental age. Though receptive vocabulary is according to mental age, comprehension of syntax lags, and they may not be able to follow or comprehend grammatical rules. Communication delays occur early in infancy, but they start responding to a person's voice by 4 months, such as typical children. But, from that point, the difference in receptive language acquisition rate diverges for infants with DS. Unlike TD infants who respond to name by 4–6 months or requests for objects by 12 months, infants with DS respond to their name between 14 and 16 months, and requests for social routines and objects by 18 months.

Few studies have shown that infants with DS tend to communicate through gestures, vocalizations, facial expressions, and other movements as TD infants do between 12 and 18 months, but for a longer period. Caselli et al. found a "gesture advantage" in young children with DS compared with matched controls for word comprehension, and despite a smaller repertoire of gestures, no differences could be found for overall usage of gestures between young children with DS and a comparison group of TD children. The gestural communication can therefore be considered a strength. On considering expressive language, a similar pattern was observed, where the first milestones were visible by 4 months for infants with DS (such as vocalizing mood and social vocalizing/laughing), but then the delay became more evident. Infants with DS start atypical vocalizing from 2 to 12 months. In the first 6 months of life, infants with DS also produce more non-speech-like sounds than speech-like sounds, which impairs the later development of normal vocal behavior. A delay in the age of onset of canonical babbling (consonant-vowel) has been found in infants with DS. Decreased vocal imitation in DS has been shown to be associated with lower expressive and receptive language skills. Acquiring first words tends to be delayed too, appearing, on average, between 18 and 36 months. Expressive vocabulary increases with developmental age in DS, as is observed in TD children. However, fewer words are produced by young children with DS when compared to children at similar overall developmental levels.

This has been demonstrated in a recent study by Onnivello et al., where infants with DS had mastered gestures as well as first vowel–consonant combinations at 14–16 months for the most part, and they uttered first words after 18 months, which is in line with previous studies on language development in DS. So, ultimately, adolescents and adults with DS have articulation problems and speech intelligibility as a major challenge. But, their prowess in gestural and nonverbal communication can come as great help to navigate their daily lives. This thus stresses the need for institutionalizing early language intervention and speech therapy in DS.

COGNITIVE MILESTONES

It has been demonstrated that performances on cognitive scale items were relatively more like those observed in TD development. Typical infants generally shift attention, prefer novel objects, explore objects, and have persistent reach by 4 months. Infants with DS also showed the same in the first 4 months, except for persistent reaching, which appeared to be mastered in the age range of 8–9 months. The initial signs of object permanence that is searching for a missing object are acquired at 6–8 months normally, but it takes another 4 months in the DS. Likewise, infants with DS find a hidden object after 18 months, unlike the TD infant, who usually does it by 1 year. It might be possible that, just as for motor development, cognitive development in early infancy is slightly delayed in DS relative to TD infants (1- or 2-month delay), but, after the 12th month, the delay in development increases in relation to the typical infants.

Older individuals with DS have shown strengths in visuospatial processing, in particular, visual memory, visual-motor integration, and especially visual imitation; though their verbal processing skills may be poor. The importance of congenital ear/auditory problems in DS lies in the fact that these causes may lead to an auditory processing disorder in DS, which in turn leads to poor auditory working memory but better visual memory. The visuospatial processing and visuoconstructive tasks may also be weak.

But, we must differentiate between auditory perception and short-term/working memory for auditorily presented information, as Jarrold et al. have identified a short-term memory deficit for auditorily presented verbal information in older individuals that cannot be blamed on sensory deficits. Infants with DS show similar event-related brain potential morphology, visual attention, and visual fixation to TD infants. Infants with DS also have faster information processing and visual imitation skills like TD infants. But unfortunately, this is not true in all areas of visuospatial functioning, and Andrews reports that 6-month-old infants with DS show delays in visual exploration in play situations with their mothers, they may also have impaired visual attention performance on a habituation task and delays in various aspects of eye contact. These early development findings also suggest that in both infancy and later development, a combination of strengths and weaknesses can be found within this area of functioning.

Delineating cognitive and communication milestones in DS may also facilitate the detection of early risk factors for a child's development. The incidence of autism spectrum disorders (ASD) is 18–40% in individuals with DS. As in TD children, features of ASD may be evident in the first 2 years of life; poor eye contact, poor response to name call, solitary play, poor nonverbal response skills which are so unlike in DS or the onset of repetitive behavior all should be watched for due to the increased incidence of ASD in DS. The most important differentiating factor here being the child with DS will be unlike its normal cheerful self, and there would not be the classical smiling face of DS if there is ASD. Challenges with attention and hyperactivity have been found in approximately 40% of school-age children with DS. In DS, attention and hyperactivity symptoms during very early development are less well understood, as they already have executive function deficits and inattention.

SOCIOEMOTIONAL MILESTONES

Almost all the delays and deficits are overcome by the socioemotional milestones of individuals with DS. An individual with DS can form lasting friendships, reciprocal nomination in the friendship dyad, convergence between parental and child nomination, and at least 6-month stability of friendship in that dyad. Children with DS are more empathetic than other children with developmental disabilities and are capable of a social response when faced with a distressing situation. They learn to compensate using their social skills. As infants and children, they smile more.

The visual imitative competence demonstrated in infancy has been described as evidence of "an innate social competence". Infants with DS look longer at their mothers than TD infants, even at 4 months of age, a behavior that may promote social connections. Other evidence of social competence in infancy can be found in increased melodic sounds, vocalic sounds, and emotional sounds in 4-month-old infants with DS when interacting with people rather than with objects. These children start to respond to maternal requests by 17.5 months such as TD children. By around 2 years of age, they display all the stranger reactions that a TD child shows when separated from his/her caregiver. Toddlers and preschoolers with DS have nonverbal social interaction, including more play acts, turn taking, invitations, and object shows compared to TD children. One major aspect of social-emotional functioning in DS that is particularly interesting is the ability to communicate positive affect through frequent emotion displays such as smiles.

Locatelli et al. had done a study in 2021 whereby the timing of certain developmental milestones may help predict the ultimate development. Observing developmental patterns in DS is informative and provides useful information to contextualize an individual's performance. They studied the timing of sitting, babbling, sphincter control, and the relation between the future attainment of complex milestones. For preschoolers, sitting was seen to be a significant predictor of later gross motor development, both assessed directly or indirectly through parent reports of everyday life behaviors. Therefore, the earlier a child with DS started to sit, the earlier he/she started to walk, run, and have stronger leg muscles that allow him/her to jump and have better general coordination or balance. Sitting also predicts future communication. In fact, being seated permits deeper breathing and more consistent subglottal pressure than a supine position. And keeping the head upright alters the position of the spine and the vocal tract curve, and the tongue falls to a more forward position in the oral cavity. This, in turn, enhances the production of consonant-vowel (CV) segments. Considering language milestones, in preschoolers, babbling showed a moderate correlation to later everyday life communication, while in school-age participants, it moderately correlated with later communication and cognition. Considered together with other developmental milestones, it emerged to be one of the significant predictors of later verbal cognitive development. In school-age children, sphincter control resulted as a significant predictor of later motor, cognitive, communication, adaptive behavior, and motor development.

An easy reckoner for the development in DS is noted in **Table 2**.

TABLE 2: Development in Down syndrome (DS)—easy reckoner.

Milestones	*Down syndrome range*	*Typical range*
Gross motor:		
Sits alone	6–30 months	5–9 months
Crawls	8–22	6–12 months
Stands	1.3–2.5 years	8–17 months
Walks alone	1–4 years	9–18 months
Language:		
First word	1–4 years	1–3 months
2-word phrases	2–7.5 years	15–32 months
Personal/Social:		
Responsive smile	1.5–5 months	1–3 months
Finger feeds	10–24 months	7–14 months
Drinks from a cup (unassisted)	12–32 months	9–17 months
Feeds with spoon	10–39 months	12–20 months
Bowel control	2–7 years	16–42 months
Dresses self (unassisted)	3.5–8.5 years	3.25–5 years

Source: File:Milestones DS.jpg. [online] Available from https://www.physio-pedia.com/index.php?title=File:Milestones_DS.jpg&oldid=185111 [Last accessed April, 2025].

CONCLUSION

Early identification is an important contributor to effective early intervention. In neurodevelopment conditions such as DS, the initial comprehensive characterization of early phenotypic profiles is essential to facilitate early identification of additional risk and for the development of new interventions and treatments. There is definitely a dire need to compare DS children with other DS children, as the incidence of ASD and Attention-Deficit/Hyperactivity Disorder (ADHD) in DS can then be easily picked up. Parents and clinicians should be aware that in addition to medical surveillance, the developmental follow-up, identification of other neurodevelopmental comorbidities, and early intervention and required therapy are needed in a child with DS. All children will require timely physiotherapy to help with hypotonia and ligamentous laxity, thus overcoming their motor deficits. They will require occupational therapy, which, in addition to improving their fine motor skills and activities of daily living, also helps to build their attention and executive function. Speech and oro-motor exercises are the most important because they will need consistent and persistent input to work on their speech and vocabulary.

SUGGESTED READING

1. Chapman RS, Hesketh LJ, Kistler DJ. Predicting longitudinal change in language production and comprehension in individuals with Down syndrome. J Speech Lang Hear Res. 2002;45(5):902-15.
2. Contestabile A, Fila T, Ceccarelli C, Bonasoni P, Bonapace L, Santini D, et al. Cell cycle alteration and decreased cell proliferation in the hippocampal dentate gyrus and in the neocortical germinal matrix of fetuses with Down syndrome and in Ts65Dn mice. Hippocampus. 2007;17(8): 665-78.
3. das Neves Cardoso AC, de Campos AC, Dos Santos MM, Santos DC, Rocha NA. Motor performance of children with Down syndrome and typical development at 2 to 4 and 26 months. Pediatric Phys Ther. 2015;27(2):135-41.
4. DiGuiseppi C, Hepburn S, Davis JM, Fidler DJ, Hartway S, Lee NR, et al. Screening for autism spectrum disorders in children with Down syndrome: population prevalence and screening test characteristics. J Dev Behav Pediatr. 2010; 31(3):181-91.
5. Dmitriev V. Early Education for Children with Down Syndrome: time to begin. Pro-Ed; 2001.
6. Fabbretti D, Pizzuto E, Vicari S, Volterra V. A story description task in children with Down's syndrome: lexical and morphosyntactic abilities. Journal of intellectual disability research. 1997;41(2).
7. Fidler DJ. The emerging Down syndrome behavioral phenotype in early childhood: Implications for practice. Infants Young Child. 2005;18(2):86-103.
8. Frank K, Esbensen AJ. Fine motor and self-care milestones for individuals with Down syndrome using a retrospective chart review. J Intellect Disabil Res. 2015;59(8):719-29.
9. Golden JA, Hyman BT. Development of the superior temporal neocortex is anomalous in trisomy 21. J Neuropathol Exp Neurol. 1994;53(5):513-20.
10. Grieco J, Pulsifer M, Seligsohn K, Skotko B, Schwartz A. Down syndrome: Cognitive and behavioral functioning across the lifespan. Am J Med Genet C Semin Med Genet. 2015;169(2):135-49.
11. Gueant JL, Anello G, Bosco P, Gueant-Rodriguez RM, Romano A, Barone C, et al. Homocysteine and related genetic polymorphisms in Down's syndrome IQ. J Neurol Neurosurg Psychiatr. 2005;76(5):706-9.
12. Harris SR, Shea AM. Down syndrome. Pediatr Neurol Phys Ther. 1991:131-68.
13. Hodapp RM, Burack JA, Zigler E (Eds). Issues in the Developmental Approach to Mental Retardation. Cambridge University Press; 1995.
14. Iverson JM, Longobardi E, Caselli MC. Relationship between gestures and words in children with Down's syndrome and typically developing children in the early stages of communicative development. Int J Lang Commun Disord. 2003;38(2):179-97.
15. Jarrold C, Baddeley AD, Hewes AK. Genetically dissociated components of working memory: Evidence from Downs and Williams syndrome. Neuropsychologia. 1999;37(6):637-51.
16. Jobling A. Motor development in school-aged children with Down syndrome: a longitudinal perspective. Int J Disabil Dev Educ. 1998;45(3):283-93.
17. Kaat-van den Os DT, Volman C, Jongmans M, Lauteslager P. Expressive vocabulary development in children with Down syndrome: a longitudinal study. J Pol Pract Intellect Disabil. 2017;14(4):311-8.
18. Karrer JH, Karrer R, Bloom D, Chaney L, Davis R. Event-related brain potentials during an extended visual recognition memory task depict delayed development of cerebral inhibitory processes among 6-month-old infants with Down syndrome. Int J Psychophysiol. 1998; 29(2):167-200.
19. Kasari C, Freeman SF, Bass W. Empathy and response to distress in children with Down syndrome. J Child Psychol Psychiatr. 2003;44(3):424-31.
20. Kim HI, Kim SW, Kim J, Jeon HR, Jung DW. Motor and Cognitive Developmental Profiles in Children with Down Syndrome. Ann Rehabil Med. 2017;41(1):97-103.
21. Klein JA, Haydar TF. Neurodevelopment in Down syndrome: Concordance in humans and models. Front Cell Neurosci. 2022;16:941855.
22. Layton T. Developmental Scale for Children with Down Syndrome. Durham, NC: Extraordinary Learning Foundation; 2004.
23. Legerstee M, Bowman TG, Fels S. People and objects affect the quality of vocalizations in infants with Down syndrome. Early Develop Parent. 1992;1(3):149-56.
24. Liogier d'Ardhuy X, Edgin JO, Bouis C, De Sola S, Goeldner C, Kishnani P, et al. Assessment of cognitive scales to examine

memory, executive function and language in individuals with Down syndrome: Implications of a 6-month observational study. Front Behav Neurosci. 2015;9:300.

25. Locatelli C, Onnivello S, Antonaros F, Feliciello A, Filoni S, Rossi S, et al. Is the age of developmental milestones a predictor for future development in Down syndrome? Brain Sci. 2021;11(5):655.
26. Lynch MP, Oller DK, Steffens ML, Levine SL, Basinger DL, Umbel V. Onset of speech-like vocalizations in infants with Down syndrome. Am J Ment Retard. 1995;100(1): 68-86.
27. McCann B, Levman J, Baumer N, Lam MY, Shiohama T, Cogger L, et al. Structural magnetic resonance imaging demonstrates volumetric brain abnormalities in Down syndrome: Newborns to young adults. Neuroimage Clin. 2021;32:102815.
28. Onnivello S, Schworer EK, Daunhauer LA, Fidler DJ. Acquisition of cognitive and communication milestones in infants with Down syndrome. J Intellect Disabil Res. 2023;67:239-53.
29. Oxelgren UW, Myrelid Å, Annerén G, Ekstam B, Göransson C, Holmbom A, et al. Prevalence of autism and attention-deficit-hyperactivity disorder in Down syndrome: a population-based study. Dev Med Child Neurol. 2017;59(3): 276-83.
30. Schmidt-Sidor B, Wisniewski KE, Shepard TH, Sersen EA. Brain growth in Down syndrome subjects 15 to 22 weeks of gestational age and birth to 60 months. Clin Neuropathol. 1990;9(4):181-90.
31. Tarui T, Im K, Madan N, Madankumar R, Skotko BG, Schwartz A, et al. Quantitative MRI analyses of regional brain growth in living fetuses with Down syndrome. Cereb Cortex. 2020;30(1):382-90.
32. Trezise KL, Gray KM, Sheppard DM. Attention and vigilance in children with Down syndrome. Journal of Applied Research in Intellectual Disabilities. 2008;21(6):502-8.
33. Tudella E, Pereira K, Basso RP, Savelsbergh GJ. Description of the motor development of 3–12-month-old infants with Down syndrome: The influence of the postural body position. Res Dev Disabil. 2011;32(5):1514-20.
34. Vicari S, Bellucci S, Carlesimo GA. Visual and spatial long-term memory: differential pattern of impairments in Williams and Down syndromes. Dev Med Child Neurol. 2005;47(5):305-11.
35. Weisz JR, Yeates KO. Cognitive development in retarded and nonretarded persons: Piagetian tests of the similar structure hypothesis. Psychol Bull. 1981;90(1):153.
36. Zampini L, D'Odorico L. Lexical and syntactic development in Italian children with Down's syndrome. Int J Lang Commun Disord. 2011;46(4):386-96.
37. Zampini L, Fasolo M, D'Odorico L. Characteristics of maternal input to children with Down syndrome: a comparison with vocabulary size and chronological age-matched groups. First Lang. 2012;32(3):324-42.

SECTION 2

Systemic Manifestations

CHAPTER 6

Congenital Heart Disease in Down Syndrome: Special Considerations

Sonia Karapurkar, Balu Vaidyanathan, Krishna Kumar R

INTRODUCTION

Congenital heart diseases (CHDs) are known to be present in about 60% children with Down syndrome (DS) in India. There are variations in the pattern of cardiac involvement in studies reported from across the globe. The most common lesion associated with DS is atrioventricular septal defect (AVSD), followed by ventricular septal defect (VSD), ostium secundum atrial septal defect (ASD), tetralogy of Fallot (TOF), and isolated patent ductus arteriosus (PDA) as per the western literature. However, VSD was found to be the most common, followed by AVSD and then ASD and PDA as per a study reported from Kerala, India. Pulmonary outflow tact obstruction lesions such as TOF and critical pulmonary stenosis are found more commonly in Asian children. Transposition of great arteries, coarctation of aorta, and left-sided obstructive lesions are few of the lesions seldom associated with DS.

Studies had identified the region D21S55 to the telomere, comprising of 4–5 Mb region, comprising of about 30 genes that may be responsible for CHDs. Further molecular mapping studies have identified five "critical regions" (DSCR1 to DSCR5), of which DSCR1 is thought to influence cardiac development, especially the valve formation and inhibition of cardiac hypertrophy. The region was identified to extend from D21S3 (defined by VSDs) through to PFKL (defined by TOF), containing 39 human genes and 25 predicted genes that are responsible for the various CHD phenotypes. Overexpression of one of these genes, DSCAM, which mediated cell-cell adhesion and epithelial-mesenchymal transformation of endocardial cushion cells, leads to various endocardial cushion defects. Further, specific gene variants or modifiers like cysteine rich with epidermal growth factor like domains (CRELD1) (3p25.1) have been identified as a locus for AVSD. Also, the folate pathway is postulated to be involved, and the reduced folate carrier (SLC19A1) was found to be associated with AVSD using a multilocus allele-sharing test.

GENERAL PHYSIOLOGICAL DERANGEMENTS

Recent studies have shown that functional cardiac abnormalities, especially ventricular diastolic dysfunction, secondary to altered myocardial fibrillar structure are present, even in anatomically normal hearts with DS. Abnormal growth of pulmonary vasculature predisposing to pulmonary hypertension and autonomic nervous system instability are also associated. Diastolic dysfunction occurs due to impaired relaxation of cardiac muscles. Increased cardiac mass is noted, likely secondary to increased expression of DSCR1, which encodes MICPI (myocyte-enriched calcineurin-interacting protein I) which inhibits calcineurin-mediated transcriptional responses that induce apoptosis of cardiac myocytes. This increased cardiac mass also contributes to diastolic dysfunction. Left ventricular (LV) hyperkinesia is reflected by increased values of ejection fraction, MAPSE (mitral annular planar systolic excursion) and mitral Sa velocity. This hyperkinesia is postulated to be a result of reduced afterload as against intrinsic myocardial abnormalities. Children with DS are known to have statistically, but not clinically significant low systolic and diastolic blood pressures (12 percentile lower than age and height-matched controls). MicroRNA hsa-miR-155 located on chromosome 21 differentially interacts with type 1 angiotensin receptor II gene, causing its under-expression, resulting in low blood pressures. However, the myocardial performance index, which combines the systolic and diastolic performance, and is independent of arterial pressure, heart rate, ventricular geometry, and preload, is found to be increased in children with DS, predominantly due to an increased isovolumic relaxation time, implying an overall decreased cardiac contractility.

Children with DS exhibit a blunted tachycardic response to orthostatic stress along with blunted sympathetic activation, vagal withdrawal, and a lesser reduction in baroreceptor sensitivity to standing. This overall impairment in autonomic cardiac regulation explains the chronotropic incompetence during exercise seen in these children. This chronotropic incompetence explains the higher incidence of cardiovascular disease and increased cardiovascular risk in these patients. The anatomic substrate for the overall impaired autonomic responses in DS is provided by the failure of growth and maturation of the brain with loss of neurons and dendrites, and damage to the neurotransmitter system as a result of the genetic disorder.

Pulmonary hypertension is known to have a higher incidence and a faster progression in children with DS. The lungs of children with DS have a smaller number of alveoli in relation to the acini (between 58 and 83% of expected number), enlarged alveolar ducts. Upregulation of the COL6A1 (collagen type VI alpha 1 chain) located on chromosome 21 is postulated to be responsible for the decreased branching and poor alveolar growth. Epigenetic modifications such as hypermethylation of the HOXB cluster are known to play a critical role in upper airway manifestations such as macroglossia, adenotonsillar hypertrophy, laryngomalacia, and tracheomalacia. Increased expression of pericentrin causes ciliopathy and increased mucous production, predisposing to repeated lower respiratory tract infections. Increased expression of the calcineurin pathway causes alveolar smooth muscle hypertrophy and modulates expression of surfactant genes. Also, the upregulation of antiangiogenetic genes like COL18A1, amyloid-beta precursor protein and DSCR1, along with decreased growth of pulmonary vasculature, contribute to pulmonary hypertension.

Obstructive sleep apnea is seen in 30–50% of children with DS as against 3% prevalence in general population. Other conditions such as gastroesophageal reflux disease and diaphragmatic hernia are more common in DS. These factors further contribute to worsening of pulmonary hypertension and overall cardiac functions in these patients. These alterations are likely to contribute to higher morbidity, length of hospital stay, and cost utilization in these patients.

SCREENING FOR CONGENITAL HEART DISEASE IN DOWN SYNDROME: PRENATAL AND POSTNATAL

The CHDs are seen in 40–50% of fetuses with DS, as against about 1% of non-DS fetuses. In healthcare systems with an access to obstetric ultrasound, a fetal echo is recommended for all pregnancies with a suspected DS. A fetal echo incorporating the necessary views as per standard practice guidelines by experienced personnel can diagnose up to 90% of CHDs. Timely identification of a complex CHD with DS may influence parental decision of continuing the pregnancy, while detection of a critical CHD can help plan immediate neonatal care.

A four-chamber view of the fetal heart is a part of most obstetric scans. Complete AVSDs, with large atrial and inlet VSDs, may demonstrate an obvious deficiency at the level of the crux of the heart. A detailed fetal echo can confirm the diagnosis, give accurate anatomical details of septal defects, AV valve morphology, and valve insufficiency. Partial AVSDs and other shunt lesions (ASD and VSD) seen in DS may be challenging, and small defects may be missed.

The prenatal detection rate of TOF is reported to be 15–43.1% in general population. The discrepancy in sizes of the great vessels, with pulmonary artery likely to be smaller than the aorta on a three-vessel view is an important diagnostic clue, but may be overlooked, and the diagnosis is likely to be missed unless a LV outflow tract view demonstrating the septoaortic discontinuity is seen in the fetal echo. TOF with hypoplastic pulmonary arteries, though seen rarely in children with DS, is a critical CHD and prenatal diagnosis can help plan immediate neonatal care.

Since the detection rate of these specific anomalies on routine prenatal scans is not very high, most guidelines recommend a dedicated fetal echo in case of a suspected DS on first or second-trimester screening. A detailed fetal echo has been shown to have a negative predictive value of 100% for complex CHDs, defined as those with RACHS category 3 and above (risk adjustment for surgery for CHD) and a 71% for other minor CHDs.

Most of the babies with DS may not display overt signs of cardiac involvement at birth regardless of the severity of the underlying CHD. Clinical examination and basic diagnostic tests like chest X-ray and ECG may have poor sensitivity and specificity in diagnosing CHDs at the hands of primary healthcare providers. Thus, echocardiographic screening is justified for all babies born with DS for early diagnosis of CHD. Early diagnosis can help in proactive management of CHD, before worsening of PAH into irreversible pulmonary vascular disease that may preclude corrective cardiac surgeries. Routine echocardiographic screening for all babies with DS is recommended by American Academy of Pediatrics.

TABLE 1: Recommendations on individual congenital heart defects in Down syndrome.

Cardiac lesion	*Special considerations*	*Recommendation*
Ventricular septal Defect (VSD)	VSD is the commonest lesions in DS. Large unrestrictive defects present with typical symptoms; pulmonary vascular disease may develop early if unoperated upon	Early corrective surgery ideally between the age of 3–6 months; earlier if clinical condition merits or later if patient presents late and is still operable. Small VSDs can be followed up
Atrial septal defects	Small secundum ASDs are common and found in association with other lesions; small defects (<8 mm) often close spontaneously	• Ostium primum defects are discussed below under AVSD • Isolated secundum defects that are large (>10 mm) should be managed electively like patients without DS
Atrioventricular septal defect (AVSD)	AVSD is almost as common as VSD. Can be partial (primum ASD alone or with restrictive VSD). Complete forms progress to becoming inoperable pulmonary vascular obstructive disease if not operated upon	• Early corrective surgery for complete AVSD after comprehensive assessment; ideally between the age of 3–6 months • Partial AVSD may be operated on an elective basis. Complex forms of AVSD such as unbalanced defects are rare and may be palliated
Patent ductus arteriosus (PDA)	Large PDAs can be missed unless carefully looked for during echocardiography	Closure is recommended ~3 months age. Catheter closure with device is often feasible
Tetralogy of Fallot	Common in DS; Presentation dictated by severity of right ventricular outflow (RVOT) obstruction	Corrective surgery recommended ~6 months age. Selected centers may offer correction early but, in the event, early correction is not feasible, palliation through BT shunt, PDA stenting, balloon pulmonary valvotomy or stenting of the RVOT may be undertaken
Combination of lesions	Common examples include TOF with AVSD (Tet-canal); VSD with PDA	Treatment strategies need to be individualized depending on the specifics of the anatomy and capability of the center
Complex situations	Examples include TOF with small or disconnected pulmonary arteries; Unbalanced AV canal, complex anatomic variants of AV canal	These can be difficult to treat and it may only be possible to offer palliation. In general, single ventricle palliation through the Fontan operation is not considered for DS patients because of concerns of high pulmonary vascular resistance

Specific considerations in management of individual category of lesions for DS are given in **Table 1**.

The DS does not pose an increased risk of mortality or long-term morbidity for congenital cardiac surgeries as compared to non-DS children for all lesions except single ventricle repairs. Chances of postoperative infections, length of hospital stay, and need for ventilation postoperative may be more in DS as compared to non-DS children, and this may be attributed to immune dysregulation and other nonimmune predisposing factors such as airway and ear abnormalities, increased predisposition to gastroesophageal reflux, etc. A comprehensive assessment and appropriate management of these factors can make most cardiac lesions in DS easily correctable with surgery or transcatheter device closures. Atlantoaxial instability and smaller airway should be taken into consideration during the preoperative anesthesia evaluation. Challenging intubation and extubation, and difficulty in weaning from the ventilator are known in this population, owing to smaller airways, and a higher incidence of airway obstruction and subglottic stenosis. About 12% children with DS undergoing cardiac surgeries are known to require prolonged ventilation postoperatively, likely due to increased incidence of pulmonary hypertension in this cohort. Increased incidence of bradycardia following anesthesia, especially with sevoflurane and dexmedetomidine is known in these children. Increased incidence of fever, due to higher levels of proinflammatory cytokines following surgery, is known in this cohort.

Children with DS with shunt lesions such as ASD and VSD present at a younger age with significant PAH as compared to non-DS children, while those with AVSD or TOF may present at similar age of their non-DS counterparts. However, they all present with lower weight than non-DS children. Incidence of requiring preoperative pulmonary artery banding or pulmonary vasodilators is higher in children with DS. A few cardiac conditions are truly challenging in them. They are rare and include unbalanced AVSD and TOF with hypoplastic pulmonary arteries. It may be only possible to palliate them or manage them medically.

Atrioventricular septal defect being the most common cardiac lesion in these children, repair of complete AVSD is the most performed surgery. Complete AVSD is more commonly seen than partial or transitional AVSD, along with associated defects like additional ASD or VSD, aortic arch obstruction, bilateral SVC, necessitating additional operative procedures such as ductus arteriosus ligation, closure of an additional VSD, aortic arch repair, and venous baffles. However, patients with DS have a lower rate of left AV valve dysplasia (3%, in DS, 24% in non-DS), unbalanced ventricles (3% in DS, 25% in non-DS), and left-sided obstructive lesions (1% in DS, 30% in non-DS). Given the additional increased risk of development of PAH in DS, early surgical repair of complete AVSD between 3 and 6 months is considered ideal. Age at repair lower than 2.5 months was found to be associated with a higher risk of mortality. Partial or transitional AVSDs, including ostium primum ASDs may be repaired electively. Unbalanced AVSDs are rare and may be palliated as appropriate.

The VSDs are the second most common lesions and present earlier in these children due to earlier development of PAH. Early corrective surgery by 3–6 months for large VSDs presenting with increased pulmonary blood flow is recommended before the onset of increased pulmonary vascular resistance. Preoperative PAH is higher in children with DS and may require pulmonary vasodilators.

Ostium secundum ASDs are quite common and managed like those with non-DS children. Preoperative PAH is significantly higher in children with DS with ASD as compared to children without DS. These children may require preoperative pulmonary vasodilators. Small defects may close spontaneously. Transcatheter closures may be done in appropriate cases, with results similar to non-DS children.

Tetralogy of Fallot is the most common cyanotic heart disease in children with DS. As with children without DS, the presentation is dictated by the severity of right ventricular outflow tract (RVOT) obstruction. Corrective surgery by 6 months of age is recommended, like in non-DS children, and in case of severely reduced pulmonary blood flow, palliative procedures such as ductus arteriosus or RVOT stenting, or aortopulmonary shunts may be undertaken until definitive repair. Repair with trans-annular patch may have a higher morbidity in DS due to inherent pulmonary vascular issues resulting in higher pulmonary vascular resistance. Hence, it is desirable to maintain competence of the pulmonary valve (PV) in surgical repair of TOF in DS by valve sparing techniques or use of valved conduits.

In single ventricle physiology, Fontan repair is now being increasingly offered to these children, however, increased incidence of pulmonary hypertension may preclude cavopulmonary shunts in these patients unless timely pulmonary banding has prevented pulmonary over circulation. Long-term pulmonary complications can significantly impact the functioning of Fontan circuit in DS predisposing to Fontan failure and its complications.

Outcomes After Surgery/Catheter Procedures: Early and Late; A Summary of Published Data

Complete balanced AVSD repairs are one of the most performed surgeries in children with DS with overall favorable outcomes. Owing to lesser variability in the AV valve morphology, rate of reoperations for left AV valve, which is the highest predictor of long-term mortality, are lower in this cohort, however, appropriate long-term follow-up is still advisable. Growth failure, with lower preoperative average weights is seen, and though some children may catch up post operatively, poor catch up growth postoperatively is also reported (27% in DS, 7% in non-DS).

Other shunt closures such as ASD and VSD surgical closures have similar outcomes in children with or without DS, apart from the requirement of preoperative pulmonary vasodilators. The risk of postoperative heart block following VSD surgical or transcatheter closure is higher in children with DS. ASD closures have similar outcomes in both groups and may prevent the early development of obstructive pulmonary hypertension in these children.

Tetralogy of Fallot repairs have overall favorable immediate and short-term outcomes. However, the incidence of PV replacement post TOF repair is higher in children with DS, likely due to increased incidence of PAH in this group. Sullivan et al. found a statistically significant greater degree of PV regurgitation on CMR in children with DS 10 years post-TOF repair, with a higher rate of RV dilatation and a lower LV ejection fraction (LVEF). Freedom from PV replacement was lower in children with DS than those without DS. Increased incidence of LV dysfunction has been seen in these children post-TOF repair as compared to non-DS children.

Outcomes with single ventricle repairs with Fontan surgery, continue to be poor in this cohort. Though significant improvement in outcomes has been reported in recent literature, morbidity and mortality continue to be significantly high.

SPECIAL CHALLENGES IN LOW RESOURCE ENVIRONMENTS

Children with DS require a holistic approach right from their birth, addressing the complications arising due to involvement of multiple systems. In lower and middle economic countries, dedicated specialized CHD services are often concentrated in urban areas. Lack of uniform availability of such centers leads to delayed diagnosis, lack of appropriate intensive care services, and decreased access to corrective cardiac surgeries. Prenatal diagnosis or neonatal screening is often limited, and children are diagnosed mainly based on phenotypic and clinical features. This leads to late presentation when they may already be inoperable due to pulmonary hypertension. A thorough evaluation of the late presenters with echocardiography, oxygen saturation, and if required, cardiac catheterization, may still identify the small proportion of the late presenters that may benefit from surgery. Infrastructure to be able to direct these patients to the specialized cardiac care centers is crucial for their definitive management, in order to reduce the burden of those with a guarded prognosis.

Education of primary care teams on the neonatal screening, and where possible, prenatal screening can help in early diagnosis from the peripheries, and the identified cohort can be offered timely management at the specialized centers. Prenatal screening for DS using nuchal translucency (NT) screening and biochemical markers should be offered to all high-risk pregnancies, especially when the maternal age is higher. Education on regular oxygen saturation monitoring, correct interpretation of the chest X-ray and ECG can help the primary care givers monitor these patients and refer to specialized centers at the right time. Establishment of referral centers, telemedicine facilities, etc., can provide support to the local teams caring for these children, to optimize outcomes. Addressing of societal factors, cultural beliefs and the stigma that is still associated with DS, via local healthcare workers in native languages may help bring out parental concerns and address them rightly to prevent undertreatment of these children.

Further, financial constraints may also negatively impact the care of these children. Providing financial resources through nongovernment organizations and charitable institutions may help more children with DS and CHD seek appropriate medical care. Government programs like Rashtriya Bal Swasthya Karyakram (RBSK) and Mahatma Jyotirao Phule Jan Arogya Yojana (MJPJAY) in India have revolutionized the availability of health care resources.

Parental education and awareness are critical in ensuring appropriate care and follow-up.

COUNSELING

Adequate parental education and sensitization of caregivers are pivotal in delivery of holistic care. Parental counseling should involve the necessity of multidisciplinary approach. A comprehensive and honest discussion with between the treating team and the family members regarding the family background, socioeconomic status, and the willingness to treat, is central to providing long-term care to these patients.

Surgical correction of the underlying CHD may often not be the endpoint in the treatment of children with DS with a CHD. Contribution of factors such as immune dysregulation, upper airway anomalies such as macroglossia, adenotonsillar hypertrophy, laryngomalacia and tracheomalacia, gastroesophageal reflex disease, atlantoaxial instability, etc., should be taken into consideration at each step, formulating an individualized management plan based on these. Regular screening for pulmonary hypertension is imperative in preoperative as well as postoperative period. Noncardiac comorbidities should be assessed as per protocols. Adequate thyroid hormone replacement, management of obstructive sleep apnea and type II respiratory failure, dental hygiene, and treatment of nutritional anemia are cornerstones for good surgical outcomes and long-term follow-up. Exercise capacity, symptoms of coronary artery disease, and adverse effects of long-term medications should be monitored subsequently.

Guidance to appropriate clinics like otorhinolaryngology, gastroenterology, immunology, etc., is crucial to handle the respective complications which may interfere with long-term surgical outcomes. Life expectancy of children with DS is now increasing, and increased awareness regarding long-term complications of cardiac surgeries in DS is required. Complications arising from primary cardiac surgeries like heart block following VSD repair, or increased incidence of PV replacement following TOF repairs must be adequately addressed with prior planning.

Superimposed issues such as learning difficulties, behavioral disorders, and early-onset dementia can make it difficult for the patients to convey their symptoms or to adhere to an appropriate lifestyle. Awareness of the available resources, and considerate planning can make it easier for the caregivers to deal with these challenging situations. The long-term aspects following cardiac surgeries should be discussed with parents or caregivers, keeping them well aware of the complications likely to arise in future.

Children with DS run a lifelong risk of LV dysfunction, and regular exercise with healthy lifestyle becomes important for weight management, cardiovascular fitness and has been shown to have beneficial effects on autonomic function. Appropriate transitional care should be offered as they transition into adulthood. Many centers treating CHDs offer care for the adult congenital heart, but where necessary an appropriate transition into the grown-up congenital heart (GUCH) clinics must be offered to these children. Assessment of decision-making capacity as they become adults is necessary and where appropriate, a surrogate decision maker must be identified as a part of advanced care planning.

Strengthening of peripheral healthcare resources with appropriate training in fields concerning care of patients with DS with CHD can help equitable distribution of care for these patients from all areas in the low socioeconomic countries.

CONCLUSION

The higher risk of postoperative morbidity and complications posed by DS are mainly related to increased risk of pulmonary hypertension and propensity to infections, along with extracardiac factors such as upper airway obstruction. DS does not pose an increased risk for cardiac surgeries and procedures as compared to children without DS as long as attention to specific details are made. Cardiac management can be successfully carried out in these children with due attention to these complicating factors. Comprehensive and holistic care with adequate parental education can minimize complications and optimize outcomes.

SUGGESTED READING

1. Abdelrahman EG, Kamal NM, Alharthi S, Albalawi M, Assar E. Down syndrome patients with normal hearts: are they really normal? Medicine (United States). 2023;102(6): e32886.
2. Al-Biltagi M, Serag AR, Hefidah MM, Mabrouk MM. Evaluation of cardiac functions with Doppler echocardiography in children with Down syndrome and anatomically normal heart. Cardiol Young. 2013;23(2):174-80.
3. Al-Biltagi MA. Echocardiography in children with Down syndrome. World J Clin Pediatr. 2013;2(4):36.
4. American Academy of Pediatrics. Committee on Genetics. American Academy of Pediatrics: Health supervision for children with Down syndrome. Pediatrics. 2001;107(2): 442-9.
5. American Institute of Ultrasound in Medicine. AIUM practice guideline for the performance of fetal echocardiography. J Ultrasound Med. 2013;32(6):1067-82.
6. Atz AM, Hawkins JA, Lu M, Cohen MS, Colan SD, Jaggers J, et al. Surgical management of complete atrioventricular septal defect: Associations with surgical technique, age, and trisomy 21. J Thorac Cardiovasc Surg. 2011;141(6):1371-9.
7. Bai W, Voepel-Lewis T, Malviya S. Hemodynamic changes in children with Down syndrome during and following inhalation induction of anesthesia with sevoflurane. J Clin Anesth. 2010;22(8):592-7.
8. Balli S, Yucel IK, Kibar AE, Ece I, Dalkiran E Sen, Candan S. Assessment of cardiac function in absence of congenital and acquired heart disease in patients with Down syndrome. World J Pediatr. 2016;12(4):463-9.
9. Barbosa Santos FCG, Croti UA, De Marchi CH, Murakami AN, Brachine JDP, Borim BC, et al. Surgical treatment for congenital heart defects in down syndrome patients. Braz J Cardiovasc Surg. 2019;34(1):1.
10. Barlow GM, Chen XN, Shi ZY, Lyons GE, Kurnit DM, Celle L, et al. Down syndrome congenital Heart disease: A narrowed region and a candidate gene. Genet Med. 2001;3(2):91-101.
11. Benhaourech S, Drighil A, El Hammiri A. Congenital heart disease and Down syndrome: various aspects of a confirmed association. Cardiovasc J Afr. 2016;27(5):287.
12. Calcagni G, Calvieri C, Baban A, Bianco F, Barracano R, Caputo M, et al. Syndromic and Non-Syndromic Patients with Repaired Tetralogy of Fallot: Does It Affect the Long-Term Outcome? J Clin Med. 2022;11(3):850.

13. Carvalho JS, Axt-Fliedner R, Chaoui R, Copel JA, Cuneo BF, Goff D, et al. ISUOG Practice Guidelines (updated): fetal cardiac screening. Ultrasound Obstet Gynecol. 2023; 61(6):788-803.
14. Cooney TP, Thurlbeck WM. Pulmonary hypoplasia in Down's syndrome. N Engl J Med. 1982;307(19):1170-3.
15. Cooper A, Sisco K, Backes CH, Dutro M, Seabrook R, Santoro SL, et al. Usefulness of Postnatal Echocardiography in Patients with Down Syndrome with Normal Fetal Echocardiograms. Pediatr Cardiol. 2019;40(8):1716-21.
16. Danopoulos S, Deutsch GH, Dumortier C, Mariani TJ, Al Alam D. Lung disease manifestations in Down syndrome. Am J Physiol Lung Cell Mol Physiol. 2021;321(5):L892.
17. Delany DR, Gaydos SS, Romeo DA, Henderson HT, Fogg KL, McKeta AS, et al. Down syndrome and congenital heart disease: perioperative planning and management. J Congen Cardiol. 2021;5(1):7.
18. Dimopoulos K, Constantine A, Clift P, Condliffe R, Moledina S, Jansen K, et al. Cardiovascular Complications of Down Syndrome: Scoping Review and Expert Consensus. Circulation. 2023;147(5):425-41.
19. Donofrio MT, Moon-Grady AJ, Hornberger LK, Copel JA, Sklansky MS, Abuhamad A, et al. Diagnosis and treatment of fetal cardiac disease: A scientific statement from the American Heart Association. Circulation. 2014;129(21):2183-242.
20. Fudge JC, Li S, Jaggers J, O'Brien SM, Peterson ED, Jacobs JP, et al. Outcomes Following Congenital Heart Surgery in Down Syndrome Patients: Analysis of a National Clinical Database. Pediatrics. 2010;126(2)315-22.
21. Furlong-Dillard J, Bailly D, Amula V, Wilkes J, Bratton S. Resource Use and Morbidities in Pediatric Cardiac Surgery Patients with Genetic Conditions. J Pediatr. 2018;193:139-41.
22. Galati DF, Sullivan KD, Pham AT, Espinosa JM, Pearson CG. Trisomy 21 Represses Cilia Formation and Function. Dev Cell. 2018;46(5):641-50.e6.
23. Giagkoudaki F, Dimitros E, Kouidi E, Deligiannis A. Effects of exercise training on heart-rate-variability indices in individuals with down syndrome. J Sport Rehabil. 2010; 19(2):173-83.
24. Hamilton J, Yaneza MMC, Clement WA, Kubba H. The prevalence of airway problems in children with Down's syndrome. Int J Pediatr Otorhinolaryngol. 2016;81:1-4.
25. Hoashi T, Hirahara N, Murakami A, Hirata Y, Ichikawa H, Kobayashi J, et al. Current Surgical Outcomes of Congenital Heart Surgery for Patients With Down Syndrome in Japan. Circulation J. 2018;82(2):403-8.
26. Iellamo F, Galante A, Legramante JM, Lippi ME, Condoluci C, Albertini G, et al. Altered autonomic cardiac regulation in individuals with Down syndrome. Am J Physiol Heart Circ Physiol. 2005 Dec;289(6):H2387-91.
27. King P, Tulloh R. Management of pulmonary hypertension and Down syndrome. Int J Clin Pract. 2011;65(SUPPL. 174): 8-13.
28. Korenberg JR, Bradleyj C, Distechet CM. Down Syndrome: Molecular Mapping of the Congenital Heart Disease and Duodenal Stenosis. Am J Hum Genet. 1992;50:294-302.
29. Lal PS, Chavan B, Devendran VR, Varghese R, Murmu UC, Kumar RS. Surgical outcome of congenital heart disease in Down's syndrome. Asian Cardiovasc Thorac Ann. 2013; 21(2):166-9.
30. Lammers AE, Stegger J, Koerten MA, Helm PC, Bauer UM, Baumgartner H, et al. Secundum type atrial septal defect in patients with trisomy 21—therapeutic strategies, outcome, and survival: A nationwide study of the German national registry for congenital heart defects. J Clin Med. 2021;10(17):3807.
31. Lee JS, Cha SG, Kim GB, Lee SY, Song MK, Kwon HW, et al. Reversibility of Pulmonary Hypertension Following Surgical Atrial Septal Defect Closure in Children with Down Syndrome. J Cardiovasc Imaging. 2019;27(4):247.
32. Locke AE, Dooley KJ, Tinker SW, Cheong SY, Feingold E, Allen EG, et al. Variation in Folate Pathway Genes Contributes to Risk of Congenital Heart Defects Among Individuals With Down Syndrome. Genet Epidemiol. 2010; 34(6):613.
33. Maslen CL, Babcock D, Robinson SW, Bean LJH, Dooley KJ, Willour VL, et al. CRELD1 mutations contribute to the occurrence of cardiac atrioventricular septal defects in Down syndrome. Am J Med Genet A. 2006;140(22):2501-5.
34. Mogra R, Zidere V, Allan LD. Prenatally detectable congenital heart defects in fetuses with Down syndrome. Ultrasound in Obstet Gynecol. 2011;38(3):320-4.
35. Morrison ML, McMahon CJ, Morrison ML, McMahon CJ. Congenital Heart Disease in Down Syndrome. Advances in Research on Down Syndrome. BMJ. 1991;302(6790):1425-7.
36. Nasser BA, Mesned AR, Mohamad T, Kabbani MS. Incidence and causes of prolonged mechanical ventilation in children with Down syndrome undergoing cardiac surgery. J Saudi Heart Assoc. 2018;30(3):247-53.
37. Olariu IC, Popoiu A, Ardelean AM, Isac R, Steflea RM, Olariu T, et al. Challenges in the Surgical Treatment of Atrioventricular Septal Defect in Children With and Without Down Syndrome in Romania—A Developing Country. Front Pediatr. 2021;9:612644.
38. Pellegrini FP, Marinoni M, Frangione V, Tedeschi A, Gandini V, Ciglia F, et al. Down syndrome, autoimmunity and T regulatory cells. Clin Exp Immunol. 2012;169(3):238.
39. Rothermel B, Vega RB, Yang J, Wu H, Bassel-Duby R, Williams RS. A protein encoded within the Down syndrome critical region is enriched in striated muscles and inhibits calcineurin signaling. J Biol Chem. 2000;275(12):8719-25.
40. Rychik J, Ayres N, Cuneo B, Gotteiner N, Hornberger L, Spevak PJ, et al. American society of echocardiography guidelines and standards for performance of the fetal echocardiogram. J Am Soc Echocardiogr. 2004;17(7):803-10.
41. Santoro JD, Lee S, Mlynash M, Mayne EW, Rafii MS, Skotko BG. Diminished Blood Pressure Profiles in Children with down Syndrome. Hypertension. 2020;75(3):819-25.

42. Sarno LA, Walters HL, Bondarenko I, Thomas R, Kobayashi D. Significant Improvements in Mortality After the Fontan Operation in Children With Down Syndrome. Ann Thorac Surg. 2020;109(3):835-41.
43. Schleiger A, Miera O, Peters B, Schmitt KRL, Kramer P, Buracionok J, et al. Long-term results after surgical repair of atrioventricular septal defect. Interact Cardiovasc Thorac Surg. 2019;28(5):789-96.
44. Sullivan RT, Frommelt PC, Hill GD. Earlier Pulmonary Valve Replacement in Down Syndrome Patients Following Tetralogy of Fallot Repair. Pediatr Cardiol. 2017;38(6).
45. Ueno K, Ninomiya Y, Shiokawa N, Hazeki D, Eguchi T, Kawano Y. Dexmedetomidine is Associated with an Increased Incidence of Bradycardia in Patients with Trisomy 21 After Surgery for Congenital Heart Disease. Pediatr Cardiol. 2016;37(7):1228-34.
46. Van Velzen CL, Clur SA, Rijlaarsdam MEB, Pajkrt E, Bax CJ, Hruda J, et al. Prenatal diagnosis of congenital heart defects: accuracy and discrepancies in a multicenter cohort. Ultrasound in Obstet Gynecol. 2016;47(5):616-22.
47. Wiseman FK, Alford KA, Tybulewicz VLJ, Fisher EMC. Down syndrome—recent progress and future prospects. Hum Mol Genet. 2009;18(R1):R75.
48. Yıldırım G, Gungorduk K, Yazıcıoğlu F, Gul A, Çakar F, Çelikkol Ö, et al. Prenatal Diagnosis of Complete Atrioventricular Septal Defect: Perinatal and Neonatal Outcomes. Obstet Gynecol Int. 2009;2009:958496.
49. Zhao Y, Edington S, Fleenor J, Sinkovskaya E, Porche L, Abuhamad A. Fetal cardiac axis in tetralogy of Fallot: associations with prenatal findings, genetic anomalies and postnatal outcome. Ultrasound Obstet Gynecol. 2017; 50(1):58-62.

CHAPTER 7

Endocrine Problems in Children with Down Syndrome

Menon PSN, Vijayakumar M

INTRODUCTION

Endocrine problems are common in children with Down syndrome (DS), and their reported incidence is much higher than in the general population. These include thyroid dysfunction, short stature, gonadal dysfunction, infertility, decreased bone mass, vitamin D deficiency, propensity to overweight/obesity, and diabetes mellitus. The prevalence increases as age advances. Precise diagnostic criteria and effective management protocols do exist for some endocrine comorbidities of DS in most developed countries; however, consensus on the best clinical practice recommendations has not yet evolved for many comorbidities of DS, especially in low- and middle-income resource countries. The recent recommendations by the Indian Academy of Pediatrics (IAP) for DS children are a welcome step in this direction.

THYROID DISORDERS

Thyroid dysfunction is the most common endocrine malfunction noted in children with DS, with an earlier onset, and it is often transient. It is not related to the gender of the child, weight, and associated comorbidities. The prevalence of thyroid disorders is much more common in DS compared to the general population. Various prevalence rates ranging from 3 to 54% have been reported in children with DS in combined pediatric age groups, with a lifetime prevalence of 13–63%. A 10-year prospective Italian study reported the probability of developing hypothyroidism increasing from 7 to 24% at 10 years. The risk for the development of thyroid dysfunction increases by 10% annually, with a significant increase in transient forms. There are a few studies from various parts of India, in which hypothyroidism was noted in 13.6–31.2%, with no difference among various cytogenetic groups of DS in some. Both hypothyroidism and hyperthyroidism are described, but hypothyroidism is much more common and includes congenital and acquired thyroid disorders.

Congenital Hypothyroidism

Congenital hypothyroidism (CH) is reported to be 28–30 times more common in neonates with DS. It is seen in approximately 1% of neonates with DS, and 50% of these newborns show altered thyroid function characterized by low free thyroxine (FT4) and elevated thyroid-stimulating hormone (TSH) levels. A review of published literature showed the incidence of primary CH to be 1 in 113–141 livebirths in DS compared to 1 in 2,000–3,000 livebirths in the general population.

Some cases of CH with DS are missed on routine newborn thyroid screening programs and picked up on thyroid tests performed within the first 6 months of life. The American Academy of Pediatrics (AAP) recommends screening for CH in all newborns, and the screening test has to be repeated at 6 months, 1 year, and every year thereafter in children with DS. Many developing countries follow similar screening guidelines. There are no specific Indian guidelines for newborn thyroid screening in DS, and the general guidelines for newborns are followed. The frequency of testing needs to be increased in those with subclinical hypothyroidism (SCH). Some experts recommend an additional screen for thyroid diseases between the newborn period and 6 months of age in children (preferably at 3 months) for early detection of CH missed during newborn screening. The justification for this recommendation is that CH is an evolving disease, and many infants who were reported to be normal during newborn screening may develop CH earlier than 6 months of age, with disastrous consequences in psychomotor development.

The TSH and FT4 cut-offs used for screening CH in children with DS are the same as those for normal children. A retrospective study of 159 newborns with DS demonstrated that T4-based newborn screening may miss cases of CH, and a combined FT4 and TSH screening is preferred. The current evidence suggests an annual increase of thyroid abnormalities by 10% and transient dysfunction in about 13%. Despite these recommendations, many children with DS are missed during newborn screening for CH and are detected at a later age.

Subclinical Hypothyroidism

The incidence of SCH characterized by elevated serum TSH and normal FT4 is higher in children with DS, and this is likely to be missed in T4-based screening programs. It is reported in 25–32% children with DS. SCH is usually asymptomatic in DS and tends to be transient and self-limiting. Almost 50% of children with SCH in DS have antithyroid antibodies, and half of these may progress to overt hypothyroidism on follow-up. Nonautoimmune SCH is more common and occurs earlier than autoimmune thyroiditis in DS, indicating a probable role of the chromosomal alteration in the onset of thyroid dysfunction.

The clinical significance of SCH in DS and the need for treatment is a matter of debate. Mild improvement in motor development and height has been reported with early treatment, but follow-up at 10 years found no developmental differences in different groups in a single-center, double-blinded, randomized controlled trial. The available evidence suggests that SCH with persistent elevation of TSH levels >10 mU/mL coupled with a goiter, or presence of antithyroid antibodies, requires treatment with thyroxine, proper follow-up, and dose titration. There is a progressive deterioration of thyroid function over time as children grow up as adolescents and adults, further increasing the prevalence in long-term studies. This has been noted in children with DS in association with higher baseline TSH levels and those with autoimmunity.

Transient Hypothyroidism

The incidence of transient hypothyroidism is also higher; many of these children are likely to be off therapy by 3 years. The high frequency of TSH elevation in DS probably suggests a resetting of the hypothalamic-pituitary-thyroid axis rather than true SCH. In view of the relatively high incidence of transient hypothyroidism, trials off levothyroxine may be considered in both congenital and transient hypothyroidism, especially if the TSH elevation is mild (<10 mU/mL), and treatment with levothyroxine is recommended only if clinical symptoms are present or TSH elevation (>10 mU/mL) persists.

Etiology and Pathogenesis of Congenital Hypothyroidism

The etiology of CH does not seem to be thyroid agenesis, as most DS patients have no abnormalities in thyroid scans. Reported causes of CH are thyroid hypoplasia, thyroid ectopia, or partial agenesis.

The reasons for increase in prevalence of CH in children with DS are the following:

- Delayed maturation of the hypothalamic-pituitary-thyroid axis leading to a higher TSH level with normal FT4 and FT3 levels
- Peripheral resistance to thyroid hormones leading to inappropriate TSH secretion and release, probably of a central etiology
- TSH insensitivity and reduced TSH bioactivity

Recent studies have suggested a probable role of increased oxidative stress in patients with DS and thyroid dysfunction. The role of elements such as copper, zinc and selenium as well as enzymes such as superoxide dismutase (SOD1), phenylalanine hydroxylase, and dual specificity tyrosine-phosphorylase-regulated kinase 1 (DYRK1A) in the development of thyroid dysfunction is under evaluation.

Clinical Features and Management of Congenital Hypothyroidism

Thyroid hormones play an important role in the neurocognitive development in the newborn period and infancy. Failure of the thyroid gland to secrete adequate amounts of thyroid hormones [T4 and triiodothyronine (T3)], regardless of its etiology, as well as any delay in the diagnosis of CH, will lead to worsening of the psychomotor development and somatic growth. The early clinical manifestations of hypothyroidism are very nonspecific and sometimes overlap with that of DS, leading to delayed diagnosis or misdiagnosis of CH. Hence, it is important to do repeat screening even after a negative newborn screening at birth, preferably earlier than the usually recommended screening at 6 months, for early detection of abnormalities in thyroid function.

The association between CH with thyroid dysfunction and gastrointestinal abnormalities such as duodenal atresia, anal atresia, and Hirschsprung disease remains unclear. The current management guidelines, including dosage for levothyroxine for CH, are the same as that for non-DS children.

Acquired Hypothyroidism

Acquired hypothyroidism is also more common in DS than in the general population. Autoimmune thyroiditis (Hashimoto thyroiditis) is the most common cause of acquired hypothyroidism and is much more common than Graves' disease, another autoimmune disease affecting the thyroid in DS. The risk of developing autoimmune thyroid disorders increases with age.

Autoimmune Thyroiditis

Autoimmunity is more commonly seen with overt hypothyroidism than subclinical forms; hence, routine checking for autoimmunity is not recommended in DS children. Detection of anti-thyroperoxidase (TPO) antibodies is higher in DS compared to the general population. The detection of antithyroid antibodies, both anti-TPO and antithyroglobulin antibodies, is a good predictor for the severity of hypothyroidism. Older children with TSH levels >10 mU/mL should be evaluated for autoimmune etiology by checking TPO antibodies. Autoimmune thyroiditis in DS is characterized by less female preference, younger age at onset, lower antibody titer at diagnosis, and association with other autoimmune diseases. It requires treatment with thyroid hormone in addition to regular monitoring of thyroid function tests. Positive antithyroglobulin antibodies and anti-TPO antibodies were associated with higher odds of more severe hypothyroidism.

Hyperthyroidism

Hyperthyroidism or Graves' disease is rare in DS but more common than in the general population, with more than 100 cases reported in patients with DS globally. There are a few case reports from India with some cases initially diagnosed as SCH reverting to hyperthyroidism. Autoimmune thyroiditis may progress to Graves' disease more frequently in DS than in the general population. Most cases are detected in childhood and adolescence, and there is no gender predilection. The clinical features are similar to earlier presentation, less severe course characterized by heat intolerance, sweating, increased irritability, and weight loss, with diffuse goiter and rarely exophthalmos. Thyroid-stimulating immunoglobulin (TSI) levels are raised, and imaging confirms the diagnosis in most cases. A more frequent association with other autoimmune disorders is seen.

The course of Graves' disease is usually benign with good response to medical treatment with carbimazole or methimazole, and many of these cases will remit subsequently. Nonpharmacological modes of therapy, such as radioiodine or surgery, were rarely needed in a series from Italy, whereas iodine-131 was beneficial in those with shorter remissions or no remission after a mean period of 40 months on medical treatment in a series from Spain. Hypothyroidism is common following radioiodine therapy, and replacement therapy with levothyroxine is necessary.

GROWTH RETARDATION AND GROWTH HORMONE

Newborns with DS mostly have lower length, weight, and smaller head circumference at birth compared with control newborns. They have reduced linear growth potential with a blunted adolescent growth spurt. Thus, growth retardation is a cardinal clinical manifestation of DS beginning prenatally. It is most noticeable from the age of 6 months, and later during adolescence.

Disease-specific growth charts are helpful to monitor the growth of DS children and to detect further growth deviation due to associated comorbidities. The first DS-specific growth charts were prepared for the American population in 1998. The Centers for Disease Control and Prevention (CDC) of the USA currently recommends the use of revised growth charts. Many countries have developed their own disease-specific growth charts for DS. In a study from Sweden combining longitudinal and cross-sectional data, the mean birth length was 48 cm for both sexes and birth weight 3.0 and 2.9 kg, respectively, for boys and girls. Boys reached a final adult height of 161.5 cm and girls 147.5 cm at relatively young ages of 16 and 14 years, respectively. Head growth was impaired with an SDS of –0.5 at birth, decreasing to –2 at 4 years of age. A study from India observed significant growth retardation with length being more affected as age advanced, with body mass index (BMI) showing progressive increase with age.

Growth Hormone-Insulin-like Growth Factor 1 Axis

Short stature in DS has multiple etiologies. There is no overt deficiency of growth hormone (GH) or GH-releasing hormone (GHRH) in most studies, but it may occur secondary to pituitary or hypothalamic dysfunction.

Selective insulin-like growth factor-1 (IGF1) deficiency is seen in children with DS >2 years with disruption of IGF1 signaling. A recent study summarized the pathogenesis of short stature to impaired GHRH–GH–IGF axis function, largely due to an abnormal quantitative and qualitative competence of the hypothalamic-pituitary axis and reduced bioactivity of endogenous GH. Other comorbidities such as congenital heart disease, thyroid dysfunction, celiac disease, obstructive sleep apnea, and feeding difficulties may aggravate growth retardation.

Growth Hormone Therapy in Down Syndrome

Early trials with recombinant GH had shown that GH therapy during infancy and childhood normalizes growth velocity and improves motor skill performance in DS. However, long-term studies did not show a positive increase in final height. A recent systematic review and meta-analysis evaluated the safety and efficacy of GH therapy in DS patients and assessed the ethical aspects of GH treatment in children with DS. Treatment with GH resulted in significantly higher growth velocity in the short term, suggesting that GH therapy should be considered in the long-term management of DS children. No significant adverse effects of GH treatment have been reported, but there is a caution about the increased risk for the development of leukemia. In addition, the improvement in psychomotor development with GH therapy is a factor in decision making for GH therapy. More long-term studies are necessary to make definite recommendations. At the time of writing, GH therapy is not approved by the US Food and Drug Administration or European Medicines Agency for the treatment of short stature in children with DS.

OBESITY AND OVERWEIGHT

Children with DS are more likely to be overweight or obese than the general population without DS. The combined prevalence of overweight and obesity varied between 23 and 70% in various studies, with the prevalence of obesity alone varying from 7 to 23%. Children with DS have a much more propensity for being overweight during the pubertal years. Typically, an infant with DS is underweight initially, but obesity sets in as age advances.

The factors leading to the development of obesity in DS are not very clear. It is attributed to decreased resting energy expenditure, decreased metabolic rate, decreased physical activity, unhealthy eating habits, and hypothyroidism. Obesity-related complications include obstructive sleep apnea, hyperinsulinemia, dyslipidemia, type 2 diabetes, and gait abnormalities. Body composition analysis with dual-energy X-ray absorptiometry (DXA) scans demonstrated that children with DS have decreased lean mass index and increased fat mass index.

Children with DS, especially those who are obese, may have an increased risk for cardiovascular disease and metabolic syndrome. A study from Chandigarh showed significantly higher leptin concentrations and higher indices of leptin resistance with low adiponectin levels in DS children compared to controls. Higher insulin resistance and lower adiponectin were also shown in another study, and their role as potential markers of metabolic syndrome needs further evaluation. The role of insulin resistance has not been thoroughly investigated in DS.

Overall, the prevalence of obesity leading to metabolic syndrome is higher in DS, and early preventive steps should be instituted in the young age group itself to prevent metabolic syndrome. Clinical evaluation and monitoring of BMI are advised in children with DS beginning at 2 years of age. Evaluation of obese children includes monitoring fasting blood glucose, fasting lipid profile, liver function tests, and glycosylated hemoglobin (HbA1C). These children and their families need appropriate counseling on lifestyle, diet, and physical activities.

GONADAL FUNCTION, PUBERTY, AND FERTILITY

Undescended Testes

Children with DS have a high incidence of cryptorchidism (6.5%), and ascending or acquired forms are common. Since there is a high chance for tumor development in DS children and testicular malignancy in cryptorchid testes, these children should be referred to pediatric surgeons early.

Hypogonadism

Primary gonadal deficiency is a well-known feature of DS; it is progressive from birth to adolescence and clearly manifests in adulthood. Children with DS have a higher level of follicle-stimulating hormone (FSH) and luteinizing hormone (LH) compared to age-matched normal children, suggesting mild hypergonadotropic hypogonadism. This is progressive from birth to adolescence, often with delayed pubertal development. This is due to some amount of Sertoli and Leydig cell dysfunction in boys and ovarian dysfunction in girls. Boys with DS have lower total testosterone levels compared with controls due to Leydig cell dysfunction owing to the excess copy of genetic material of chromosome 21. Barring this, the onset of puberty is not much delayed in these children, and the majority of them will have normal pubertal progression. The disease-specific growth charts show that children with DS have a decreased pubertal growth spurt. Girls will need education regarding care during menstrual cycles, management of dysmenorrhea, and premenstrual symptoms.

In many cases, sex hormone levels are not very low, indicating their capacity to be fertile, and many married DS adults have children. In general, men with DS have lower fertility, but 70% of women with DS are fertile. The chances of miscarriage are higher. There is a 50% chance of having a child with DS and a higher chance of having other congenital anomalies. Hence, these children and their parents should be counseled properly about the issues in puberty, potential for fertility, and precautions to be adopted when these children are nearing adolescence.

DIABETES MELLITUS

Children with DS have a higher prevalence of diabetes mellitus than the general population. Both type 1 and type 2 diabetes have been reported in children with DS.

Type 1 Diabetes Mellitus

Type 1 diabetes is seen in around 2% of children with DS, with a 4-fold increase in the risk for development of type 1 diabetes compared with the general population of the same age. An earlier onset of type 1 diabetes in DS than general population is noted in some studies. Type 1 diabetes in DS is associated with increased subclinical islet cell autoimmunity with a lower frequency of the high-risk *HLA* genes. Type 1 diabetes in DS is also linked with other autoimmune diseases, mainly autoimmune thyroiditis and celiac disease. The expression of *AIRE* gene is also reduced in DS patients. These children usually have a better metabolic control despite lower insulin doses and lower rates of diabetes-related complications.

Type 2 Diabetes Mellitus

The reported prevalence of type 2 diabetes in children with DS ranges between 0 and 3.6%. The incidence increased with age, BMI, family history, and in girls, as shown in a report from Hyderabad. The association of type 2 diabetes in DS seems to be linked to sedentary lifestyle, obesity and metabolic diseases, and peripheral insulin resistance with declining β-cell function. Principles of management are the same as in the general population—lifestyle modification, weight loss, and oral antidiabetic drugs. The metabolic consequences of DS with type 2 diabetes require further validation.

DISORDERS OF BONE HEALTH

Defective bone strength with increased fragility and osteoporosis, leading to frequent fractures, is a common problem in DS. This is mainly due to faulty bone mineral accrual due to deficient intake of calcium and vitamin D. Lack of proper sun exposure, sedentary habits, poor muscle mass, malabsorption, and antiepileptic use are some of the etiological factors attributed to reduced bone mineral density (BMD) in these children. The bone mass of DS children may be exaggerated by the abnormalities in anthropometry and body composition. In addition, associated health issues such as developmental disorders, hypotonia of muscles, hypogonadism, growth retardation, and thyroid dysfunction may affect bone health.

There are very few studies that have evaluated the bone health and vitamin D status in DS. Some studies have evaluated bone density using dual-energy X-ray absorptiometry (DXA), peripheral quantitative computed tomography (pQCT), or quantitative ultrasound (QUS). Children with DS have lower BMD compared to healthy controls, especially of the lumbar spine. There are no recommendations for periodic BMD scans in DS children as of now; however, it seems reasonable to do periodic scans in high-risk groups such as those with obesity, hypotonia, neuromuscular disability, or abnormal metabolic parameters.

There are only a few studies that have evaluated the vitamin D status by estimating 25-hydroxyvitamin D [25(OH)D] in children with DS, but the results are conflicting. A study from Italy demonstrated a high prevalence of vitamin D deficiency in all age groups of DS. The few studies about biochemical bone markers or the prevalence of fractures are not conclusive. More studies are needed, especially from the developing world. Ensuring proper vitamin D supplementation, calcium-containing diet (milk and milk products), regular weight-bearing exercises, and encouraging outdoor play for proper sun exposure will improve bone health in children with

DS. There are no specific recommendations for vitamin D supplementation for DS. Current practice for vitamin D supplementation to prevent vitamin D deficiency is the same as for the general population.

AUTOIMMUNE DISORDERS

Children with DS are much more prone to autoimmune disorders such as type 1 diabetes mellitus, celiac disease, vitiligo, and alopecia areata, especially in the presence of autoimmune thyroiditis. The mechanism underlying the high frequency of autoimmune diseases in DS is not clearly established. The increased incidence of autoimmune disease in DS has been hypothesized to be attributable to:

- Altered immune function in DS, either humoral or cellular
- Mutations in the autoimmune regulator (*AIRE*) gene located in the 21q22.3 region, which regulates T-cell function and self-recognition, by coding for a transcription factor necessary for expression of tissue-restricted antigens (TRAs) in thymic epithelial cells
- Alterations in the regulation of pro- and anti-inflammatory cytokines
- The suppressive effect of interferon-alpha and its toxic effect on the thyroid gland
- Association with the DQA1 0301 allele linked to the increased association of autoimmune thyroid disease and celiac disease

There are no clear recommendations for routine screening for autoimmune disorders in children with DS.

Celiac Disease

Celiac disease is a common autoimmune disorder caused by gliadin and related proteins of wheat. It is very commonly seen in association with other autoimmune disorders and DS, the symptomatic form being more common than the asymptomatic. Studies have noted 6–10-fold increase in risk of developing CD for DS patients compared to the general population and affecting up to 7% of the DS children and GH deficiency. Nearly half of the children with CD do not have recognized symptoms, leading to a possibility of missed or delayed diagnoses. The European Societies for Pediatric Gastroenterology, Hepatology, and Nutrition (ESPGHAN) recommend screening all children with DS after age 3 years, and earlier if symptoms are apparent. The AAP, however, recommends only symptom-based screening from age 1. The significance of detecting CD early is its association with hypothyroidism, GH deficiency, type 1 diabetes, and other hormonal disorders, both in DS and the general population.

OTHER CHRONIC SYSTEMIC DISORDERS

Children with DS with CH are at increased risk of developing congenital anomalies, especially congenital heart diseases and gastrointestinal anomalies, compared to patients with DS and without CH. The inter-relationships of these disorders with endocrine comorbidities are being evaluated.

CONCLUSION

Current research has helped us to understand the pathophysiology and management of endocrine disorders associated with DS in children, which can impact their health and development. Thyroid dysfunction is common in individuals with DS, and early periodic screening is essential. Controversy remains regarding the treatment of SCH given unclear benefits. The use of disease-specific growth charts needs to be encouraged. There is no clear evidence to suggest routine GH therapy in DS children. Puberty develops normally in individuals with DS, and fertility is possible. Both obesity and overweight are common. Further research is needed in the field of BMD in DS. The pathophysiologic mechanism for the increase in autoimmune diseases is better understood now. There is a need to screen for both type 1 and type 2 diabetes. The efforts of the healthcare providers should be channeled to improve the life expectancy for individuals with DS and provide better opportunities to optimize medical management to reduce morbidity and maximize function.

SUGGESTED READING

1. Amr NH. Thyroid disorders in subjects with Down syndrome: an update. Acta Biomed. 2018;89(1):132-9.
2. Annerén G, Gustavson KH, Sara VR, Tuvemo T. Growth retardation in Down syndrome in relation to insulin-like growth factors and growth hormone. Am J Med Genet Suppl. 1990;7:59-62
3. Anwar AJ, Walker JD, Frier BM. Type 1 diabetes mellitus and Down's syndrome: prevalence, management and diabetic complications. Diabet Med. 1998;15(2):160-3.
4. Araya P, Kinning KT, Coughlan C, Smith KP, Granrath RE, Enriquez-Estrada BA, et al. IGF1 deficiency integrates stunted growth and neurodegeneration in Down syndrome. Cell Rep. 2022;41(13):111883.
5. Aversa T, Salerno M, Radetti G, Faienza MF, Iughetti L, Corrias A, et al. Peculiarities of presentation and evolution over time of Hashimoto's thyroiditis in children and

adolescents with Down's syndrome. Hormones. 2015; 14(3):410-6.

6. Basil JS, Santoro SL, Martin LJ, Healy KW, Chini BA, Saal HM. Retrospective study of obesity in children with Down syndrome. J Pediatr. 2016;173:143-8.
7. Bergholdt R, Eising S, Nerup J, Pociot F. Increased prevalence of Down's syndrome in individuals with type 1 diabetes in Denmark: A nationwide population-based study. Diabetol. 2006;49(6):1179-82.
8. Bertapelli F, Pitetti K, Agiovlasitis S, Guerra-Junior G. Overweight and obesity in children and adolescents with Down syndrome-prevalence, determinants, consequences, and interventions: a literature review. Res Dev Disabil. 2016;57:181-92.
9. Binder ND. Growth hormone therapy in children with Down syndrome. J Pediatr. 1992;120(5):832-3.
10. Blethen SL. Leukemia in children treated with growth hormone. Trends Endocrinol Metab. 1998;9(9):367-70.
11. Bull MJ; Committee on Genetics. Health supervision for children with Down syndrome. Pediatrics. 2011;128(2): 393-406.
12. Butler AE, Sacks W, Rizza RA, Butler PC. Down syndrome-associated diabetes is not due to a congenital deficiency in β cells. J Endocr Soc. 2017;1(1):39-45.
13. Campos C, Casado A. Oxidative stress, thyroid dysfunction & Down syndrome. Indian J Med Res. 2015;142(2):113-9.
14. Chew G, Hutson JM. Incidence of cryptorchidism and ascending tastes in trisomy 21: A 10 year retrospective review. Pediatr Surg Int. 2004;20(10):744-7.
15. Cronk C, Crocker AC, Pueschel SM, Shea AM, Zackai E, Pickens G, et al. Growth charts for children with Down syndrome: 1 month to 18 years of age. Pediatrics. 1988;81(1): 102-10.
16. Dayal D, Jain P, Panigrahi I, Bhattacharya A, Sachdeva N. Thyroid dysfunction in Indian children Down syndrome. Indian Pediatr. 2014;51(9):751-2.
17. De Luca F, Corrias A, Salerno M, Wasniewska M, Gastaldi R, Cassio A, et al. Peculiarities of Graves' disease in children and adolescents with Down syndrome. Eur J Endocrinol. 2010;162(3):591-5.
18. Dittmar M, Kahaly GJ. Immunoregulatory and susceptibility genes in thyroid and polyglandular autoimmunity. Thyroid. 2005;15(3):239-50.
19. Erlichman I, Mimouni FB, Erlichman M, Schimmel MS. Thyroxine-based screening for congenital hypothyroidism in neonates with Down syndrome. J Pediatr. 2016;173:165-8.
20. Fernhoff PM, Brown AL, Elsas LJ. Congenital hypothyroidism: increased risk of neonatal morbidity results in delayed treatment. Lancet. 1987;1(8531):490-1.
21. Ferrari M, Stagi S. Autoimmunity and genetic syndromes: A focus on Down syndrome. Genes (Basel). 2021;12(2):268.
22. Ferry B, Gavris M, Tifrea C, Serbanoiu S, Pop AC, Bembea M, et al. The bone tissue of children and adolescents with Down syndrome is sensitive to mechanical stress in certain skeletal locations: a 1-year physical training program study. Res Dev Disabil. 2014;35(9):2077-84.
23. Fonseca CT, Amaral DM, Ribeiro MG, Beserra IC, Guimarães MM. Insulin resistance in adolescents with Down syndrome: a cross-sectional study. BMC Endocr Disord. 2005;5:6.
24. Garcia-Hoyos M, Riancho JA, Valero C. Bone health in Down syndrome. Med Clin (Barc). 2017;149(2):78-82.
25. Gibson PA, Newton RW, Selby K, Price DA, Leyland K, Addison GM. Longitudinal study of thyroid function in Down's syndrome in the first two decades. Arch Dis Child. 2005;90(6):574-8.
26. Gillespie KM, Dix RJ, Williams AJ, Newton R, Robinson ZF, Bingley PJ, et al. Islet autoimmunity in children with Down's syndrome. Diabetes. 2006;55(11):3185-8.
27. Gimenez-Barcons M, Casteras A, Armengol M del P, Porta E, Correa PA, Marín A, et al. Autoimmune predisposition in Down syndrome may result from a partial central tolerance failure due to insufficient intrathymic expression of AIRE and peripheral antigens. J Immunol. 2014;193(8): 3872-9.
28. Goday-Arno A, Cerda-Esteva M, Flores-Le-Roux JA, Chillaron-Jordan JJ, Corretger JM, Cano-Pérez JF. Hyperthyroidism in a population with Down syndrome (DS). Clin Endocrinol (Oxf). 2009;71(1):110-4.
29. González-Agüero A, Vicente-Rodríguez G, Gómez-Cabello A, Casajús JA. Cortical and trabecular bone at the radius and tibia in male and female adolescents with Down syndrome: a peripheral quantitative computed tomography (pQCT) Study. Osteoporosis Int. 2013;24(3):1035-44.
30. González-Agüero A, Vicente-Rodríguez G, Moreno LA, Casajús JA. Bone mass in male and female children and adolescents with Down syndrome. Osteoporosis Int. 2011; 22(7):2151-7.
31. Graber E, Chacko E, Regelmann MO, Costin G, Rapaport R. Down syndrome and thyroid function. Endocrinol Metab Clin North Am. 2012;41(4):735-45.
32. Hsiang YH, Berkovitz GD, Bland GL, Migeon CJ, Warren AC. Gonadal function in patients with Down syndrome. Am J Med Genet. 1987;27(2):449-58.
33. Iughetti L, Predieri B, Bruzzi P, Predieri F, Vellani G, Madeo SF, et al. Ten-year longitudinal study of thyroid function in children with Down's Syndrome. Horm Res Paediatr. 2014;82(2):113-21.
34. John ST, Gayathri K, Ahmed S, Multtani KS, Menon PSN, Kumar RK, et al. Consensus statement of the Neurodevelopmental Pediatrics Chapter of Indian Academy of Pediatrics (IAP) on the management of children with Down syndrome. Indian Pediatr. 2023;60(4):298-307.
35. John ST, Gayathri K, Sahasranam KV. Cytogenetic patterns, congenital heart disease, and thyroid dysfunction in children with Down syndrome. J Pediatr. 2022;245:196-200.
36. Karlsson B, Gustafsson J, Hedov G, Ivarsson SA, Annerén G. Thyroid dysfunction in Down's syndrome: Relation

to age and thyroid autoimmunity. Arch Dis Child. 1998; 79(3):242-5.
37. Kennedy RL, Jones TH, Cuckle HS. Down's syndrome and the thyroid. Clin Endocrinol (Oxf). 1992;37(6):471-6.
38. Khan SH, Mahajan A, Rather TA. Radioactive iodine-131 as a definitive treatment in rare association of Down syndrome with hyperthyroidism: A case report and review of literature. Indian J Nucl Med. 2017;32(1):19-24.
39. King K, O'Gorman C, Gallagher S. Thyroid dysfunction in children with Down syndrome: a literature review. Ir J Med Sci. 2014;183(1):1-6.
40. Kota SK, Tripathy PR, Kota SK, Jammula S. Type 2 diabetes mellitus: an unusual association with Down's syndrome. Indian J Hum Genet. 2013;19(3):358-9.
41. Lagan N, Huggard D, Mc Grane F, Leahy TR, Franklin O, Roche E, et al. Multiorgan involvement and management in children with Down syndrome. Acta Paediatr. 2020;109(6): 1096-111.
42. Liu E, Wolter-Warmerdam K, Marmolejo J, Daniels D, Prince G, Hickey F. Routine screening for celiac disease in children with Down syndrome improves case finding. J Pediatr Gastroenterol Nutr. 2020;71(2):252-6.
43. Marchal JP, Maurice-Stam H, Ikelaar NA, Klouwer FC, Verhorstert KW, Witteveen ME, et al. Effects of early thyroxine treatment started in the neonatal period on development and growth at age 10.7 years: Follow-up of a randomized placebo-controlled trial in children with Down's syndrome. J Clin Endocrinol Metab. 2014;99(12): E2722-9.
44. Matute-Llorente A, González-Agüero A, Gómez-Cabello A, Vicente-Rodríguez G, Casajús JA. Decreased levels of physical activity in adolescents with Down syndrome are related with low bone mineral density: a cross-sectional study. BMC Endocr Disord. 2013;13:22.
45. Metwaalley KA, Farghaly HS. Endocrinal. dysfunction in children with Down syndrome. Ann Pediatr Endocrinol Metab. 2022;27(1):15-21.
46. Meyerovitch J, Antebi F, Greenberg-Dotan S, Bar-Tal O, Hochberg Z. Hyperthyrotropinemia in untreated subjects with Down's syndrome aged 6 months to 64 years: A comparative analysis. Arch Dis Child. 2012;97(7):595-8.
47. Moreau M, Benhaddou S, Dard R, Tolu S, Hamzé R, Vialard F, et al. Metabolic diseases and Down syndrome: How are they linked together? Biomedicines. 2021;9(2):221.
48. Mortimer GL, Gillespie KM. Early onset of autoimmune diabetes in children with Down syndrome-two separate aetiologies or an immune system pre-programmed for autoimmunity? Curr Diab Rep. 2020;20(9):47.
49. Mulu B, Fantahun B. Thyroid abnormalities in children with Down syndrome at St. Paul's hospital millennium medical college, Ethiopia. Endocrinol Diabet Metab. 2022;5:e00337.
50. Munns CF, Shaw N, Kiely M, Specker BL, Thacher TD, Ozono K, et al. Global consensus recommendations on prevention and management of nutritional rickets. J Clin Endocrinol Metab. 2016;101(2):394-415.
51. Murray J, Ryan-Krause P. Obesity in children with Down syndrome: background and recommendations for management. Pediatr Nurs. 2010;36(6):314-9.
52. Myrelid Å, Bergnan S, Elfvik Strömberg M, Jonsson B, Nyberg F, Gustafsson J, et al. Late effects of early growth hormone treatment in Down syndrome. Acta Paediatr. 2010;99(5):763-9.
53. Myrelid A, Jonsson B, Guthenberg C, Annerén G. Growth charts for Down's syndrome from birth to 18 years of age. Arch Dis Child. 2002;87(2):97-103.
54. Narayanan DL, Yesodharan D, Kappanayil M, Kuthiroly S, Thampi MV, Hamza Z, et al. Cardiac spectrum, cytogenetic analysis and thyroid profile of 418 children with Down syndrome from South India: a cross sectional study. Indian J Pediatr. 2014;81(6):547-51.
55. O'Grady MJ, Cody D. Subclinical hypothyroidism in childhood. Arch Dis Child. 2011;96(3):280-4.
56. Pascanu I, BanescuC, Benedeck T, Duicu C, Csep K, Dema A. Thyroid dysfunction in children with Down's syndrome. Acta Endocrinologica (Buc). 2009;5(1):85-92.
57. Pavlovic M, Berenji K, Bukurov M. Screening for celiac disease in Down syndrome – Old and new dilemmas. World J Clin Cases. 2017;5(7):264-9.
58. Pepe G, Corica D, de Sanctis L, Salerno M, Faienza MF, Tessaris D, et al. Prospective evaluation of autoimmune and non-autoimmune subclinical hypothyroidism in Down syndrome children. Eur J Endocrinol. 2020;182(3):385-92.
59. Pierce MJ, LaFranchi SH, Pinter JD. Characterization of thyroid abnormalities in a large cohort of children with Down syndrome. Horm Res Paediatr. 2017;87(3):170-8.
60. Piro E, Pennino C, Cammarata M, Corsello G, Grenci A, Lo Giudice C, et al. Growth charts of Down syndrome in Sicily: evaluation of 382 children 0-14 years of age. Am J Med Genet Suppl. 1990;7:66-70.
61. Pradhan M, Dalal A, Khan F, Agrawal S. Fertility in men with Down syndrome: A case report. Fertil Steril. 2006;86(6):1765.e1-3.
62. Prasher V, Haque MS. Misdiagnosis of thyroid disorders in Down syndrome: time to reexamine the myth? Am J Ment Retard. 2005;110(1):23-7.
63. Priya MP, Gupta N, Nagori A, Lodha R, Jain V, Pandey RM, et al. Physical growth and its determinants in Indian children with Down syndrome, from 3 months to 5 months of age. Indian J Pediatr. 2022;89(2):141-7.
64. Purdy JB, Singh N, Brown WL, Vangala S, Devaskar UP. Revisiting early hypothyroidism screening in infants with Down syndrome. J Perinatol. 2014;34(12):936-40.
65. Reza SM, Rasool H, Mansour S, Abdollah H. Effects of calcium and training on the development of bone density in children with Down syndrome. Res Dev Disabil. 2013; 34(12):4304-9.

66. Rivkees S, Bauer AJ. Thyroid disorders in children and adolescents. In: Sperling MA, Majzoub JA, Menon RK, Stratakis CA (Eds). Sperling Pediatric Endocrinology, 5th edition; 2021.
67. Rohrer T, Hennes P, Thon A, Dost A, Grabert M, Rami B, et al. Down's syndrome in diabetic patients aged <20 years: an analysis of metabolic status, glycaemic control and autoimmunity in comparison with type 1 diabetes. Diabetologia. 2010;53(6):1070-5.
68. Sankar VS, Anjukrishna K, Riaz I. Thyroid stimulating hormone level at diagnosis as a predictor of persistent subclinical hypothyroidism in children with Down syndrome. Indian Pediatr. 2018;55(7):576-8.
69. Shaki D, Hershkovitz E, Tamam S, Bollotin A, David O, Yalovitsky G, et al. GH treatment in pediatric Down syndrome: a systematic review and mini meta-analysis. Front Endocrinol (Lausanne). 2023;14:1135768.
70. Shaki D, Hershkovitz E, Tamam S, Bollotin A, David O, Yalovitsky G, et al. GHRH-GH-IGF1 axis in pediatric Down syndrome: a systematic review and mini meta-analysis. Front Pediatr. 2023;11:1132296.
71. Skogberg G, Lundberg V, Lindgren S, Gudmundsdottir J, Sandström K, Kämpe O, et al. Altered expression of autoimmune regulator in infant Down syndrome thymus, a possible contributor to an autoimmune phenotype. J Immunol. 2014;193(5):2187-95.
72. Stagi S, Lapi E, Romano S, Bargiacchi S, Brambilla A, Giglio S, et al. Determinants of vitamin D levels in children and adolescents with Down syndrome. Int J Endocrinol. 2015;2015:896758.
73. Tenneti N, Dayal D, Sharda S, Panigrahi I, Didi M, Attri SV, et al. Concentrations of leptin, adiponectin and other parameters in non-obese children with Down syndrome. J Pediatr Endocrinol Metab. 2017;30(8):831-7.
74. van Trotsenburg AS, Vulsma T, van Rozenburg-Marres SL, van Baar AL, Ridder JC, Heymans HS, et al. The effect of thyroxine treatment started in the neonatal period on development and growth of two-year-old Down syndrome children: a randomized clinical trial. J Clin Endocrinol Metab. 2005;90(6):3304-11.
75. van Trotsenburg ASP, Vulsma T, van Santen HM, Cheung W, de Vijlder JJM. Lower neonatal screening thyroxine concentrations in Down syndrome newborns. J Clin Endocrinol Metab. 2003;88(4):1512-5.
76. Whooten R, Schmitt J, Schwartz A. Endocrine manifestations of Down syndrome. Curr Opin Endocrinol Diabetes Obes. 2018;25(1):661-6.
77. Wu J. Bone mass and density in preadolescent boys with and without Down syndrome. Osteoporosis Int. 2013; 24(11):2847-54.
78. Yahia S, El-Farahaty R, El-Gilany A, Shoaib R, Ramadan R, Salem N. Serum adiponectin, body adiposity, and metabolic parameters in obese Egyptian children with Down syndrome. J Pediatr Endocrinol Metab. 2021;34(11): 1401-10.
79. Zemel BS, Pipan M, Stallings VA, Hall W, Schadt K, Freedman DS, et al. Growth charts for children with Down syndrome in the United States. Pediatrics. 2015;136(5): e1204-11.

CHAPTER 8

Growth Monitoring

Riya Lukose

INTRODUCTION

For any child, the measurement of his/her growth and development assessment is of primordial importance. Up-to-date growth charts are therefore necessary for evaluation of physical growth and for providing optimal health care. The World Health Organization has produced a global standard chart describing how children, under optimal conditions, grow worldwide, thus implying that all humans are similar in nature. But growth patterns do differ according to racial and ethnic backgrounds, and there have therefore been regional modifications, and ultimately, healthcare workers prefer to use growth charts of a well-defined reference group related to the population where they work.

Similarly, in conditions like Down syndrome (DS), Turner syndrome, etc. where it has been known to affect growth, syndrome-specific growth charts have been provided. One of the first DS-specific growth charts that have been introduced is the Centers for Disease Control and Prevention (CDC) charts in 1988 from the United States of America (USA). This was followed by various other countries. In 2002, Myrelid et al. published growth charts of DS from 1–18 years in Swedish population, which showed that Swedish adults with DS, though shorter than their peers, were taller than their American counterparts. Styles et al. from the United Kingdom (UK) compared developmental patterns in terms of body weight, height, and head circumference in children with DS to children without DS. Appreciable differences were noted for body weight, which indicates the difference in the initial weight of children with DS compared to those without DS. Reference values are thus essential for assessing linear growth. However, as many older children and adults with the syndrome are overweight, the reference values for weight should not be used as a standard that children should aim to achieve. Body mass index (BMI) information is included on the charts, particularly, to aid the assessment of those who may be overweight.

GROWTH CHARTS

The DS growth charts have been researched in North-West India by Bhalla et al. where children with DS (1–10 years) were compared to their normal Multicentric Growth Reference Study (MGRS) and Indian counterparts; the children with DS had lower weight and height attainments. The boys and girls with DS showed short stature (height < third centile) from the age of 1 year till 10 years. As compared to their normal counterparts, children with DS exhibited compromised auxological attainments.

The initial growth in a child with DS is known to lag behind their peers, especially in the first 2 years; it may be due to their inherent low growth capacity or maybe due to associated conditions like sucking/swallowing difficulties due to muscle hypotonia, oromotor dysfunction or associated cardiac conditions or gastrointestinal abnormalities. The short stature in DS can also be caused by deficiencies in growth hormone and insulin-like growth factor-1 (IGF-1) as well as zinc.

It has been shown that the growth retardation in DS occurs right from the intrauterine period itself till 38 weeks of gestation. Babies with DS then grow at par with their typical peers, after which the rate of weight gain slows down. But most of the time, babies with DS are born earlier (average 38 weeks), and they may take longer than other babies to get back to their birth weight. Unlike normal babies who regain their birth weight by 10th day, babies with DS may take up to 2 weeks. But if this regain takes longer than 4 weeks or if there is greater loss (>10%) of birth weight, other causes for the failure to gain weight such as cardiovascular diseases, feeding difficulties, etc. should be looked for. Even after birth, the growth velocity in DS is reduced, especially between 6 and 36 months.

After 3 years, they have a normal pattern of growth till they reach puberty, but the duration of the growth spurt is smaller. It was believed that these children will not survive for long and were not considered for corrective heart surgeries till a few decades ago. Now, through medical monitoring and follow-up, even if not meticulously performed in many countries, at least gross morbidities are picked up and treatments have been offered. Thus, children with DS grow into adulthood and their life expectancy has increased up to 60 years. Moreover, over time, the growth potential of all children has shown an increase and this could have happened to DS population too. In view of such circumstances, there arose a need for revision of the previous DS-specific growth charts. In the US the charts by Down Syndrome Growing-up Study (DSGS) growth charts are being recommended as they can be used as screening tools to assess growth and nutritional status. The DSGS growth charts were also similar to the recent UK charts. The UK Down Syndrome Charts launched in 2022 are included in the Royal College of Paediatrics and Child Health Digital Growth Chart application programme interface (API).

The DS-specific growth charts will help in the growing years to pick up any reason for growth faltering. The challenge is to choose the kind of growth charts for the assessment of a given parameter so that the obtained results have a real impact on clinical decisions. The original hypothesis assumed that DS-specific growth charts are the chief tools in the comprehensive assessment (weight, height, and BMI) of the developmental disorders in a child with DS.

WEIGHT AND BODY MASS INDEX

Having explained about the importance of monitoring the growth in DS let us look into the problems that we may face if we rigidly stick to DS-specific growth charts. Weight disorders in DS are challenging as they face undernutrition in the initial few years, which is then replaced by excessive weight gain in puberty and adulthood, and thus, they are prone to all the consequences too. The reasons for undernutrition in the initial years have already been mentioned. During this period, it is advisable to follow the DS-specific charts as we will be able to detect any falling off the centiles or plateauing of the weight, which can thus give us a clue to detect disorders that can result in undernutrition such a celiac disease, hyperthyroidism, diabetes mellitus, malabsorption, etc. As the child moves into first and second decades of life, they tend to gain weight. This may be attributed to different reasons like increased food/junk food intake, lack of exercise, hypothyroidism, etc. Therefore, depending on the age, this population is exposed to both deficiencies in nutrition as well as excess body weight and all the associated health consequences. The incidence of obesity is around 45% in DS when compared to 33% in normal counterparts, and it has been shown that the risk of atherosclerosis is not reduced in DS as previously thought; therefore, prevention and early treatment are principal aspects. Both BMI and body weight are assessed using growth charts to detect body weight disorders. Therefore, in the latter half of first decade and beyond, in an individual with DS, it is important that we pick up overweight/obesity, which may be masked when we use DS-specific growth charts where the centiles will be higher when compared to typical population.

The study by Hatch-Stein et al. showed that for individuals with DS, the 85th percentile on standard growth charts is a better indicator of excess adiposity than the 85th percentile on the DS-specific BMI growth charts and claimed that standard charts should be the preferred method for early identification of obesity in children with DS. The CDC has also concurred to this observation and stated that using a DS growth chart would give a false sense of security to individuals with DS. Hence, ideally, BMI and weight in adolescents should be plotted in standard growth charts such that measures can be taken to prevent obesity. Hetman et al., in 2022, have once again confirmed this in their study. So, the family should be educated on the need to avoid high-calorie diet, should practice dietary diversity, encourage children to be involved in daily judicious exercise, avoiding the risk-sports like football, trampoline etc., and thus prevent the augmentation of the obesity epidemic in persons with DS. So, they may require a multidisciplinary team including a physician, nutritionist, psychologist, trainer, and cardiologist for the management of obesity and its complications. A tremendous role in the whole process is played by parents and guardians. The whole family should be motivated to follow proper nutrition and activity patterns.

HEIGHT IN DOWN SYNDROME

Mean peak height velocities in Swedish males and females were 8.5 and 7.3 cm per year, respectively, and are significantly lower than in healthy children. The mean ages at peak height velocity were 12.3 and 10.8 years, respectively, indicating early growth spurts. The variability in height of individuals with DS was extensively studied in the Dutch population in 2012. Their established growth charts demonstrate mainly three age periods when height differences between children with and without DS increase—(1) during intrauterine life, (2) during the first 3 years of life, and (3) during puberty. This growth pattern results in a mean final height of 163.4 cm in healthy boys with DS and 151.8 cm in girls (which amounts to a difference of 3 SD in comparison to the general population), and mean head circumference (HC) at birth of 33 cm and 44 cm at the age of 15 months (almost 2 SD less than in the general Dutch population).

The mean age of onset of puberty was 10.3 ± 1.0 years in a study conducted in Turkey by Erdogan et al. in 2022 (10.0 ± 0.8 years for girls and 10.6 ± 1.2 years for boys). Obesity was seen in 46% of pubertal girls with DS. Menarche was detected to occur early in females with DS but breast development lags, and there is a tendency toward obesity in the whole population. While in males, the age of pubertal onset was similar to healthy children and the duration of puberty was longer in this study.

Other studies have shown that DS-specific chart suggests an absence of pubertal growth spurt. However, these children do have an adolescent growth spurt. It is usually less pronounced than in the general population and may occur at an earlier age. Final height is achieved earlier than in the general population. If early onset of puberty occurs, it may have a limiting effect on final height. The use of growth hormone in DS shows no evidence that it should be prescribed except in the unusual situation of concurrent primary growth hormone deficiency. The influence of parental height on target height appears to be variable.

CONCLUSION

When planning the growth monitoring in DS, the recommendations put forward by Down Syndrome Medical Interest Group (DSMIG) are commendable and easy to practice.

In the first 2 years of life, we can record the weight, length, and weight for height in the DS-specific growth charts; thereafter, annual recordings should be made during childhood and later. This will help anticipate any growth problems that we may encounter. The growth spurts and plateaux tend to be more prolonged in DS population. HC should be plotted at birth, at 6 weeks, and at regular intervals. Preterm babies can be recorded on standard intrauterine growth charts till term, as there are no published birth weight charts for preterm babies with DS who are born before 37 completed weeks.

Children below the 2nd centile for weight need evaluation. These may include perfectly healthy individuals or those with medical issues, but on average if they remain on the same growth centile without dropping off, they do not need expert pediatric opinion regarding supplementary feeding.

During adolescent period, it is better to look into weight and BMI in a normal chart as it is important that we pick up overweight/obesity, as mentioned earlier, which may be masked when we use DS-specific growth charts where the centiles will be higher when compared to typical population. If the growth chart for a particular population is not available, any standard chart can be used to monitor the growth pattern, but it is always preferable to use a DS-specific growth chart in the first decade of life.

SUGGESTED READING

1. Arnell H, Gustafsson J, Ivarsson SA, Annerén G. Growth and pubertal development in Down syndrome. Acta Paediatr. 1996;85(9):1102-6.
2. Bhalla AK, Kaur H, Kaur R, Panigrahi I. Growth charts for weight and height of Indian children with Down syndrome. Am J Med Genet A. 2024;194(7):e63571.
3. Cronk C, Crocker AC, Pueschel SM, Shea AM, Zackai E, Pickens G, et al. Growth charts for children with Down syndrome: 1 month to 18 years of age. Pediatrics. 1998;81(1):102-10.
4. Erdoğan F, Güven A. Is there a secular trend regarding puberty in children with Down syndrome? Front Endocrinology. 2022;13:1001985.
5. Ergaz-Shaltiel Z, Engel O, Erlichman I, Naveh Y, Schimmel MS, Tenenbaum A. Neonatal characteristics and perinatal complications in neonates with Down syndrome. Am J Med Genet A. 2017;173(5):1279-86.
6. Hetman M, Moreira H, Barg E. The best tool for the assessment of developmental disorders in children with down syndrome: Comparison of standard and specialized growth charts-cross sectional study. Front Endocrinology. 2022;13:928151.
7. Mazurek D, Wyka J. Down syndrome-genetic and nutritional aspects of accompanying disorders. Rocz Panstw Zakl Hig. 2015;66(3):189-94.

8. McCoy EE. Growth patterns in Down's syndrome. Down syndrome: Advances in Medical Care. New York: Wiley-Liss Inc; 1992.
9. Morris JK, Cole TJ, Springett, Dennis J. Down syndrome birth weight in England and Wales: Implications for clinical practice. Am J Med Genet Part A. 2015;167A(12):3070-5.
10. Myrelid A, Gustafsson J, Ollars B, Annerén G. Growth charts for Down's syndrome from birth to 18 years of age. Arch Dis Child. 2002;87(2):97-103.
11. Styles ME, Cole TJ, Dennis J, Preece MA. New cross-sectional stature, weight and head circumference references for Down's syndrome in the UK and Republic of Ireland. Arch Dis Child. 2002;87(2):104-8.
12. van Buuren S, Van Wouwe JP. WHO Child Growth Standards in action. Arch Dis Child. 2008;93(7):549-51.
13. World Health Organization (WHO) Multicentre Growth Reference Study Group. WHO Child Growth Standards based on length/height, weight and age. Acta Paediatr Suppl. 2006;450:76-85.
14. Zemel BS, Pipan M, Stallings VA, Hall W, Schadt K, Freedman DS, et al. Growth charts for children with Down syndrome in the United States. Pediatrics. 2015;136(5):e1204-11.

CHAPTER 9

Musculoskeletal Issues in Down Syndrome: A Guide for Pediatricians

Easwar T Ramani

INTRODUCTION

Down syndrome (DS), also known as trisomy 21, leads to a wide range of physical and cognitive impairments, including musculoskeletal complications. As a pediatrician, it is crucial to be well-versed in the musculoskeletal manifestations of DS to provide comprehensive care and early intervention for these individuals. The musculoskeletal system in individuals with DS is affected due to various factors such as hypotonia, ligamentous laxity, and abnormal bone and joint development. They can significantly impact mobility, functional independence, and quality of life.

This chapter aims to provide a comprehensive overview of the musculoskeletal issues associated with DS, highlighting the importance of regular screening, early intervention, and multidisciplinary management strategies.

HYPOTONIA AND LIGAMENTOUS LAXITY

Hypotonia, or low muscle tone, is one of the most common musculoskeletal features observed in individuals with DS. Hypotonia is present from birth and may persist throughout life, affecting overall muscle strength and coordination. Ligamentous laxity (loose ligaments) is another common characteristic, contributing to joint instability and an increased risk of dislocations and subluxations. The combination of hypotonia and ligamentous laxity can lead to various musculoskeletal complications:

- *Delayed motor development:* Infants and children with DS may experience delays in attaining developmental milestones due to decreased muscle tone and strength.
- *Postural abnormalities:* Hypotonia and ligamentous laxity may contribute to poor posture, slouching, and abnormal spinal curvatures (e.g., kyphosis, lordosis, and scoliosis).
- *Joint instability:* Loose ligaments around joints, such as the knees, hips, and shoulders, increase the risk of dislocations, subluxations, and sprains.
- *Foot deformities:* Ligamentous laxity and muscle imbalances may lead to various foot deformities, including flat feet (pes planovalgus), in-toeing (metatarsus adductus), and clubfoot (talipes equinovarus).

Physical therapy and occupational therapy help improve muscle strength, flexibility, and motor skills, while bracing or orthotic devices may be necessary in some cases to support joint stability.

COMMON SPINE PROBLEMS

- *Atlantoaxial instability (AAI):* AAI is the most concerning and potentially severe spinal abnormality in DS. It involves excessive mobility between the first (C1) and second (C2) cervical vertebrae due to ligamentous laxity or bony anomalies.
- *Scoliosis:* Scoliosis, a lateral curvature of the spine, is a frequent musculoskeletal manifestation, affecting up to 18% of individuals by adulthood.
- *Kyphosis:* Excessive outward curvature of the upper spine (thoracic kyphosis) is also more prevalent in individuals with DS.
- *Spondylolisthesis:* This forward slippage of a vertebra on the one below is occasionally seen.

Atlantoaxial Instability

Atlantoaxial instability is a developmental anomaly often occurring in people with DS and is a potentially serious condition. According to various reports, AAI affects from 6.8 to 27% of the population with DS. It is characterized by increased mobility or instability between the C1 (atlas) and C2 (axis) cervical vertebrae, which may lead to compression of the spinal cord. Children between 3 and 5 years are especially at risk. AAI can lead to spinal cord compression, presenting with symptoms such as neck pain, altered gait, clumsiness, changes in bowel/bladder function, or torticollis.

The following screening guidelines are recommended for AAI in individuals with DS:

- *Baseline screening:* Screening guidelines are controversial but generally (refer to screening recommendations below) do not support routine cervical spine screening for children <3 years and those with no symptoms. For children with symptoms, a single cervical spine lateral X-ray is advised, and if abnormal, flexion and extension lateral views of the cervical spine are taken. Screening is also advised for children who engage in contact sports.
- *Periodic screening:* If the initial screening is negative for AAI, some authorities recommend a periodic follow-up with clinical examination every 1–2 years until skeletal maturity is reached. Radiographs are included if there is any new symptom or neurological sign.
- *Symptom-based screening:* If an individual with DS develops new neurological symptoms (e.g., weakness, gait disturbances, neck pain, or bladder/bowel incontinence), immediate cervical spine evaluation is warranted, regardless of age.
- *Early detection and management of AAI* are crucial to prevent potentially life-threatening spinal cord compression. Treatment options include immobilization with a cervical collar or surgical stabilization, depending on the severity of the condition.

Scoliosis and Kyphosis

Scoliosis and kyphosis are common spinal deformities observed in individuals with DS. The incidence of scoliosis is higher than in the general population. The prevalence of scoliosis in individuals with DS ranges from 8 to 18%, while kyphosis is reported in up to 25% of cases. These spinal deformities may lead to cosmetic concerns, respiratory impairment, and functional limitations if left untreated. Adolescents with poorer functional level, especially lower motor functional status, are likely to develop larger scoliotic curves and present a greater risk for surgery. Regular screening for scoliosis and kyphosis is essential in individuals with DS. Milbrandt TA and Johnston CE, in their experience of 50 years with scoliosis in DS, noted that scoliosis developed in 8.7% of patients over time.

The following guidelines are recommended:

- *Clinical examination:* Regular physical examinations, including assessment of spinal curvature, should be performed at each well-child visit or annual health maintenance visit.
- *Radiographic screening:* If a spinal deformity is suspected on clinical examination, standing posteroanterior and lateral radiographs of the entire spine should be obtained for further evaluation.
- *Periodic follow-up:* If a spinal deformity is present, regular radiographic follow-up (e.g., every 6–12 months) is recommended to monitor progression.

Management of scoliosis and kyphosis in individuals with DS may involve bracing, physical therapy, or surgical intervention (e.g., spinal fusion), depending on the severity and progression of the deformity. There is a high rate of cardiac surgery within this population. Bracing was found to be ineffective for the majority of the patients, and surgery has a high rate of complications.

HIP PROBLEMS

- *Developmental dysplasia of the hip (DDH):* DS children have a higher incidence of hip dysplasia due to acetabular insufficiency, ligamentous laxity, and muscle hypotonia. Delayed diagnosis and treatment of DDH can lead to joint instability, pain, altered gait mechanics, and early-onset osteoarthritis. The inherent ligamentous laxity associated with DS predisposes children to hip dysplasia and, in more severe cases, complete hip dislocation. Hip instability significantly compromises joint function and mobility.
- *Slipped capital femoral epiphysis (SCFE):* Children and adolescents with DS are more prone to SCFE, where the epiphysis of the proximal femur slips posteromedially off the femoral neck. Symptoms often include hip or groin pain with a limp. SCFE requires urgent orthopedic intervention. The results of operative treatment are, however, guarded.
- *Legg-Calvé-Perthes disease (LCPD):* Although less common than DDH and SCFE, LCPD occurs at a higher frequency in children with DS. LCPD involves a temporary disruption of the blood supply to the femoral head. Children may present with pain, limping, and limited hip motion. The radiological features and treatment are similar to the general population.
- *Hip dysplasia and dislocation:* Hip dysplasia, or abnormal development of the hip joint, is a common

musculoskeletal condition in individuals with DS. It can range from mild hip instability to complete dislocation of the femoral head from the acetabulum.

The prevalence of hip dysplasia in individuals with DS is estimated to be around 1–7%. This can result in progressive loss of mobility and function. The etiology of hip instability is a combination of hypotonia, ligamentous laxity, and abnormal hip morphology. Early detection and management are crucial to prevent long-term complications, such as osteoarthritis, gait abnormalities, and functional limitations.

Natural history has been well described. The initial presentation in children <2 years old is delayed walking, hypotonia, and ligamentous laxity, leading to unstable hips. From ages 2 to 8 years, the hip instability may progress to dislocations that can be reduced. After the age of 8 years, hip subluxation progresses, and it cannot be concentrically reduced. There is also associated acetabular dysplasia. The final stage occurs in late adolescence or early adulthood with a fixed dislocated hip.

Even though universal screening of the hip is controversial, the following screening guidelines are recommended for hip dysplasia in individuals with DS:

- *Newborn screening:* All infants with DS should undergo a physical examination of the hips, including the Ortolani and Barlow maneuvers, within the first few weeks of life. A routine ultrasound screening of the hip can be done where feasible.
- *Radiographic screening:* If the initial physical examination is abnormal or concerning, pelvic radiographs should be obtained to evaluate for hip dysplasia or dislocation.
- *Periodic screening:* Periodic follow-up examinations and radiographs, if necessary, should be performed at regular intervals (e.g., every 6–12 months) until skeletal maturity is reached (see section below and **Table 1**). Clinical examination alone has been found to be inadequate to diagnose hip dysplasia in DS. So, radiographic evaluation is recommended until 16 years of age for early detection of hip dysplasia.

Treatment options for hip dysplasia in individuals with DS include bracing (e.g., Pavlik harness), closed reduction and spica casting, or surgical intervention (e.g., open reduction and pelvic osteotomy) in severe cases. Management depends on the phase of hip instability. For patients under age 2 years, nonoperative treatment is preferable. For older patients, the treatment is aimed at stabilizing the hip and preventing acetabular dysplasia.

COMMON KNEE PROBLEMS

- *Patellofemoral instability (PFI):* Generalized ligamentous laxity, muscle weakness, and abnormal knee alignment are key risk factors for PFI in individuals with DS. PFI can cause pain, knee "giving way", difficulty with stairs, and kneeling or squatting.
- *Genu valgum (knock knees):* Excessive genu valgum is frequently seen in DS and can contribute to PFI and altered gait mechanics.
- *Ligament injuries:* The inherent ligamentous laxity associated with DS may predispose children to various ligament injuries around the knee.
- *Inflammatory arthropathy:* This is an underdiagnosed entity and many times picked up very late in DS. This is usually part of polyarthritis with small joint predominance. Early treatment is important to prevent a significant disease burden.

Patellofemoral Instability

Patellofemoral instability, sometimes referred to as "chondromalacia patellae" or "runner's knee," refers to instability of the patella due to weak muscles, lax ligaments, or abnormal tracking of the patella within the femoral groove. While PFI can affect anyone, it is more prevalent in individuals with DS due to the underlying ligamentous laxity. Symptoms include:

- Knee pain, especially during activities such as climbing stairs or running
- Frequent knee buckling or giving way
- Difficulty in squatting or kneeling

A comprehensive physical examination, including gait analysis and assessment of patellar tracking, is needed to diagnose PFI. Imaging studies such as X-rays are basic investigations, and a child may require an MRI if symptoms are persistent.

Treatment typically involves nonsurgical approaches such as:

- *Physical therapy* to strengthen muscles and improve joint stability
- *Bracing* to support the patella
- *Activity modification* to reduce stress on the knee joint

Surgery may be considered for severe cases that fail to respond to conservative management.

FOOT DEFORMITIES

Foot deformities, such as flat feet (pes planus), in-toeing (metatarsus adductus), and clubfoot (talipes equinovarus), are commonly observed in individuals with DS due to ligamentous laxity, muscle imbalances, and abnormal bone development. The prevalence of flat feet in individuals with DS is estimated to be around 50%, while the incidence of clubfoot ranges from 1 to 7%.

Early recognition and management of foot deformities are crucial to prevent long-term complications, such as pain, gait abnormalities, and functional limitations. The following screening and management strategies are recommended:

- *Newborn screening:* All infants with DS should undergo a thorough examination of the feet and lower extremities at birth to identify any congenital deformities.
- *Periodic follow-up:* Regular follow-up examinations should be performed during well-child visits to monitor for the development or progression of foot deformities.
- *Orthotic management:* In mild cases of flat feet or in-toeing, orthotic devices (e.g., ankle-foot orthoses and shoe inserts) may be prescribed to provide support. Cases of clubfoot are treated with the Ponseti casting protocol with excellent results. Clubfeet in children with DS have similar rates of recurrence and may have better clinical outcomes when compared with their idiopathic counterparts.
- *Physical therapy:* Stretching and strengthening exercises, as well as gait training, can be beneficial in managing foot deformities and improving overall function.
- *Surgical intervention:* In severe cases of foot deformities, such as rigid clubfoot or severe flexible flat feet, surgical intervention (e.g., tendon transfers or bony procedures) may be necessary. Surgery in planovalgus foot is generally restricted to cases where the deformity is very severe or painful with callosity.

INFLAMMATORY ARTHRITIS

There is an increased predisposition to inflammatory arthritis known as Down syndrome-associated arthritis (DA). It is characterized by early onset polyarticular involvement that tends to be aggressive and results in significant joint damage at diagnosis. This is mostly due to the delay in recognition and initiation of treatment. The delay is attributed partly to the absence of formal screening guidelines for inflammatory arthritis within this population.

The average delay from symptom onset to diagnosis was 2 years in a study by Juj H et al. Prevalence of DA is 8.7/1000, more than 6 times higher than juvenile idiopathic arthritis (JIA) in the general population. Age at onset varied from 20 months to 12 years in their study. At symptom onset, 57% had polyarticular disease, and 43% had oligoarticular disease, but 54% with oligoarticular disease progressed to polyarticular disease. Most required second-line therapy, and almost half had developed joint subluxation.

The prevalence and severity of DA are not merely anecdotal but are supported by substantial clinical observations. Jones JT et al. highlighted that most individuals with DS presenting with DA have polyarticular disease activity that is both rheumatoid factor and antinuclear antibody negative at the time of diagnosis. Despite aggressive therapeutic interventions using disease-modifying antirheumatic drugs (DMARDs), management remains challenging due to medication toxicity, inefficacy concerns, and high disease burden observed among affected individuals.

The exploration by Kamalakar A et al. into aneuploidy's impact on skeletal health provides valuable insights into how chromosomal aberrations such as those seen in DS can influence bone mass and architecture, leading potentially toward altered mechanical properties that may predispose individuals with DS to various forms of arthritis, including DA. This connection between chromosomal abnormality and altered skeletal health underscores the complex interplay between genetics and musculoskeletal pathology in DS.

Most of the available literature on DA comes from observational studies or clinical reviews, which inherently possess limitations regarding causality inference and potential biases. Moreover, there exists a notable gap in large-scale epidemiological data specifically addressing the incidence rate or risk factors associated with DA development beyond generic associations drawn from smaller cohort analyses or case reports. Juj H et al. noted that the prognosis in inflammatory arthritis in children with DS is much poorer than JIA.

OSTEOPOROSIS AND FRACTURE RISK

Individuals with DS are at an increased risk of developing osteoporosis, a condition characterized by low bone mass and deterioration of bone tissue, leading to an increased susceptibility to fractures. Angelopoulou N et al. reported that the bone mineral density (BMD) of the lumbar spine in males as well as in females with DS was significantly lower than that in their control counterparts.

The underlying mechanisms contributing to osteoporosis in DS are not fully understood but may involve factors such as reduced physical activity, nutritional deficiencies, hormonal imbalances, and genetic factors. Angelopaulo N et al. studied men with DS and other intellectual deficiencies (ID) and found that BMD in individuals with DS versus young adults was lower at the 26% level (T-score –2.66 ± 0.29) and significantly lower ($p = 0.002$) than that of the ID group.

The following screening and management strategies are generally recommended for osteoporosis and fracture risk in individuals with DS:

- *Bone mineral density screening:* Regular BMD assessments using dual-energy X-ray absorptiometry (DXA) should be performed, starting in late adolescence or early adulthood, to evaluate bone health and fracture risk.
- *Nutritional assessment:* Evaluation of dietary intake and supplementation of calcium, vitamin D, and other essential nutrients may be necessary to optimize bone health.
- *Physical activity promotion:* Encouraging regular weight-bearing and muscle-strengthening exercises can help improve bone mass and reduce fracture risk.
- *Pharmacological intervention:* In cases of severe osteoporosis or high fracture risk, pharmacological interventions, such as bisphosphonates or other osteoporosis medications, may be considered under the guidance of an endocrinologist or rheumatologist.
- *Fall prevention:* Implementing strategies to reduce the risk of falls, such as environmental modifications, assistive devices, and physical therapy interventions, can help prevent fractures in individuals with DS.

SCREENING AND MANAGEMENT STRATEGIES

Effective screening and management of musculoskeletal issues in individuals with DS require a multidisciplinary approach involving pediatricians, orthopedic surgeons, physical therapists, occupational therapists, and other healthcare professionals. The following general screening and management strategies are recommended:

- *Regular screening:* Implement a comprehensive screening protocol, including physical examinations, radiographic evaluations, and specialized assessments, as outlined in this chapter.
- *Early intervention:* Prompt diagnosis and initiation of appropriate interventions, such as physical therapy, bracing, or surgical correction, can significantly improve functional outcomes and prevent long-term complications.
- *Multidisciplinary care:* Collaborate with a team of specialists, including orthopedic surgeons, physical therapists, occupational therapists, and other healthcare professionals, to develop a coordinated and comprehensive treatment plan.
- *Family education and support:* Provide education and support to families and caregivers regarding the musculoskeletal manifestations of DS, the importance of adherence to treatment plans, and strategies for promoting physical activity and functional independence.
- *Transition planning:* Ensure a seamless transition from pediatric to adult care by providing comprehensive medical records, facilitating communication with adult healthcare providers, and addressing any potential gaps in care.
- *Ongoing monitoring and follow-up:* Regularly monitor the individual's musculoskeletal status, adjust treatment plans as needed, and provide ongoing support and guidance throughout their lifespan.

Screening Guidelines

There are some standardized orthopedic screening protocols for children with DS **(Table 1)**. The major concise guidelines by various organizations are briefly discussed here.

American Academy of Pediatrics (AAP) Health Supervision Guidelines for Children with Down Syndrome

- Perform a comprehensive musculoskeletal evaluation at each well-child visit, including assessment of muscle tone, hyperreflexia, joint mobility, and spinal curvature.
- Routine radiographic screening of asymptomatic children for AAI is not recommended. A child <3 years does not have adequate vertebral mineralization and epiphyseal development for accurate radiographic evaluation of the cervical spine. Plain radiographs do not predict well which children are at increased risk of

developing spine problems, and normal radiographs do not provide assurance that a child will not develop spine problems later. Therefore, routine radiologic evaluation of the cervical spine in asymptomatic children is not recommended. For symptomatic children, obtain cervical spine radiographs. The initial radiograph should be in a neutral position. This is checked for abnormality, and if it is normal, a necessary lateral view in flexion and extension positions can be supplemented. If the neutral view itself reveals abnormalities, the child should be referred to a pediatric neurosurgeon.

- Perform hip examination (Ortolani and Barlow maneuvers) at birth and repeat at 6 weeks, 6 months, and annually until skeletal maturity is attained to screen for DDH. Obtain pelvic radiographs if hip examination is abnormal for DDH.
- Refer to appropriate specialists (e.g., orthopedic surgeon and physical therapist) for further evaluation and management as needed.

Down Syndrome Medical Interest Group (DSMIG) (UK) Health Care Guidelines

- Perform a musculoskeletal examination at each well-child visit, including assessment of muscle tone, joint mobility, spinal curvature, and foot deformities.
- Cervical spine X-ray lateral view has no predictive value in the later development of instability. Hence, a screening X-ray is not routinely recommended. However, if patient develops any new symptoms or warning signs (see list below), it is important to consider AAI as a possibility and take appropriate cervical spine X-rays and refer to a specialist. Warning signs of AAI include:
  - Neck pain
  - Abnormal head posture
  - Torticollis (wry neck)
  - Reduced neck movements
  - Deterioration of gait and/or frequent falls
  - Increasing fatigability on walking
  - Deterioration of manipulative skills
- Perform hip examination (Ortolani and Barlow maneuvers) at birth, 6 weeks, 6 months, and annually until skeletal maturity to screen for DDH. Obtain pelvic radiographs only if hip examination is abnormal or if there are risk factors for DDH. (However, Van Gijzen et al. in their study found that clinical history and physical examination are insufficient to timely detect DDH in children with DS. They recommend regular radiological examination of the hip till 16 years of age.)
- Children are prone to inflammatory arthritis. It is important to screen for the disease, especially if a child has a recent onset of poor mobility or complains of pain.
- Orthopedic diseases to be aware of in DS include the following:
  - Pes planus
  - Scoliosis, particularly post-thoracotomy
  - Craniovertebral instability
  - Cervical arthropathy
  - Lumbar spondylolysis and spondylolisthesis
  - Hip instability, including subluxation and dislocation
  - SCFE
  - LCPD
  - Osteoarthritis of the hip
  - PFI
  - Congenital talipes equinovarus (CTEV)
  - Metatarsus primus varus and associated hallux valgus and varus

MULTIDISCIPLINARY APPROACH AND TRANSITION TO ADULT CARE

The management of musculoskeletal issues in individuals with DS requires a multidisciplinary approach involving various healthcare professionals, including pediatricians, orthopedic surgeons, physical therapists, occupational therapists, and other specialists as needed. Pediatricians play a pivotal role in coordinating care and facilitating communication among the multidisciplinary team members. Regular team meetings or case conferences can help ensure that all members are aware of the individual's specific needs and treatment goals, and that care plans are consistently implemented and adjusted as necessary.

As individuals with DS transit from pediatric to adult care, it is essential to ensure a seamless transition process. Pediatricians should work closely with adult healthcare providers, such as internists, family physicians, and adult orthopedic specialists, to ensure continuity of care and to address any potential gaps in services or treatment plans. Transition planning should begin well in advance and should involve the individual with DS, their family or caregivers, and all relevant healthcare providers. This process should include the following steps:

1. *Medical summary and treatment plan:* Prepare a comprehensive medical summary, including the individual's medical history, current treatment plans, and any ongoing musculoskeletal issues or concerns.
2. *Transfer of records:* Ensure that all relevant medical records, including diagnostic reports, imaging studies, and treatment notes, are transferred to the adult healthcare providers.
3. *Communication and coordination:* Facilitate communication between the pediatric and adult healthcare teams, ensuring a thorough understanding of the individual's needs and any necessary modifications to the treatment plan.
4. *Self-care and independence:* Provide education and support to the individual with DS and their family or caregivers regarding self-care strategies, exercise programs, and the importance of adherence to treatment plans and regular follow-up visits.
5. *Community resources and support services:* Provide information about community resources, support groups, and advocacy organizations that can assist the individual and their family or caregivers during the transition to adult care.
6. *Ongoing monitoring and follow-up:* Schedule regular follow-up appointments with the adult healthcare team to monitor the individual's musculoskeletal status, adjust treatment plans as needed, and address any emerging concerns or issues.

By implementing a coordinated and comprehensive transition process, pediatricians can help ensure that individuals with DS continue to receive high-quality care and support as they navigate the transition to adult healthcare services.

TABLE 1: Summary of musculoskeletal screening timeline in Down syndrome.

Age	*Area of focus*	*Screening tests/evaluations*	*Considerations*
Birth to 6 months	Hip instability/ dysplasia	Clinical hip exam (Barlow/Ortolani maneuvers). Ultrasound if abnormalities are detected or if there are risk factors. Assess for leg length discrepancy	Early detection is essential for optimal management and preventing long-term complications
Ongoing	Developmental delays	Routine developmental assessments, including gross motor milestones	Delays in achieving milestones may necessitate further evaluation for underlying musculoskeletal or neurological conditions
6 months to 2 years	Hip instability	Follow-up if clinical concerns or risk factors persist. Consider X-rays if indicated	Continued vigilance is important, as undetected hip problems can contribute to pain and disability later in life
2 to 5 years	Atlantoaxial instability (AAI)	Cervical spine X-rays (including flexion/ extension views). MRI if instability is identified	Screening is essential, as AAI can lead to spinal cord compression if not detected early
2 to 5 years	Patellofemoral instability (PFI)	Physical exam, gait assessment. Consider imaging if there is knee pain, instability, or functional limitations	Symptoms may be subtle in young children; careful evaluation is warranted
5 years to skeletal maturity	Scoliosis	Adams forward bend test, scoliometer use	Full spine X-rays if scoliosis is detected
Throughout lifespan	Foot and ankle deformities	Routine foot examination at well-visits, including gait assessment	Flat feet (pes planus), bunions (hallux valgus), or high arches (pes cavus) can impact function and comfort
Throughout lifespan	Overall musculo-skeletal health	Assessment of joint range of motion, muscle strength, pain, and functional limitations	Generalized ligamentous laxity may predispose individuals to joint hypermobility, instability, and premature arthritis
As needed	Concerning symptoms	Prompt evaluation with targeted physical examination and imaging as indicated	New pain, changes in function, gait, bowel/ bladder function, or neurologic symptoms should be thoroughly investigated

CONCLUSION

Down syndrome is associated with a wide range of musculoskeletal complications, including hypotonia, ligamentous laxity, AAI, hip dysplasia, scoliosis, kyphosis, foot deformities, and an increased risk of osteoporosis and fractures. Early recognition, regular screening, and prompt intervention are crucial to prevent long-term complications and optimize functional outcomes. Pediatricians play a vital role in the comprehensive care of individuals with DS by implementing standardized screening protocols as shown in **Table 1**, collaborating with a multidisciplinary team of specialists, and providing education and support to families and caregivers.

This chapter also highlights the importance of a seamless transition process from pediatric to adult care, involving comprehensive medical summaries, transfer of records, effective communication and coordination among healthcare teams, and ongoing monitoring and follow-up. Through a collaborative and patient-centered approach, pediatricians can make a significant difference in the lives of individuals with DS and their families, helping them navigate the challenges of musculoskeletal complications and promoting overall health and well-being.

SUGGESTED READING

1. American Academy of Pediatrics. Committee on Genetics. American Academy of Pediatrics: Health supervision for children with Down syndrome. Pediatrics. 2001;107(2):442-9.
2. Angelopoulou N, Matziari C, Tsimaras V, Sakadamis A, Souftas V, Mandroukas K. Bone mineral density and muscle strength in young men with mental retardation (with and without Down syndrome). Calcif Tissue Int. 2000;66(3):176-80.
3. Angelopoulou N, Souftas V, Sakadamis A, Mandroukas K. Bone mineral density in adults with Down's syndrome. Eur Radiol. 1999;9(4):648-51.
4. Baptista F, Varela A, Sardinha LB. Bone mineral mass in males and females with and without Down syndrome. Osteoporos Int. 2005;16(4):380-8.
5. Bosch P, Johnston CE, Karol L. Slipped capital femoral epiphysis in patients with Down syndrome. J Pediatr Orthop. 2004;24(3):271-7.
6. Bull MJ, Trotter T, Santoro SL, Christensen C, Grout RW; THE COUNCIL ON GENETICS. Health Supervision for Children and Adolescents with Down Syndrome. Pediatrics. 2022;149(5):e2022057010.
7. Caird MS, Wills BP, Dormans JP. Down syndrome in children: the role of the orthopaedic surgeon. J Am Acad Orthop Surg. 2006;14(11):610-9.
8. Caselli MA, Cohen-Sobel E, Thompson J, Adler J, Gonzalez L. Biomechanical management of children and adolescents with Down syndrome. J Am Podiatr Med Assoc. 1991;81(3):119-27.
9. Down Syndrome Medical Interest Group (DSMIG) Health Care Guidelines. (2012). [online] Available from https://www.dsmig.org.uk/wp-content/uploads/2015/09/CSI-revision-final-2012.pdf [Last accessed April, 2025].
10. Duque Orozco MDP, Abousamra O, Chen BP, Rogers KJ, Sees JP, Miller F. Knee Deformities in Children with Down Syndrome: A Focus on Knee Malalignment. J Pediatr Orthop. 2018;38(5):266-73.
11. Egea-Gámez RM, Galán-Olleros M, Martínez-Caballero I, Ramírez-Barragán A, Serrano JI, Palazón-Quevedo Á, et al. Scoliosis in Adolescent Patients with Down Syndrome: Correlation Between Curve Magnitude and Functional Level. Clin Spine Surg. 2023;36(10):E471-7.
12. Foley C, Killeen OG. Musculoskeletal anomalies in children with Down syndrome: an observational study. Arch Dis Child. 2019;104(5):482-7.
13. Foley CM, Deely DA, MacDermott EJ, Kiileen OG. Arthropathy of Down syndrome: an under-diagnosed inflammatory joint disease that warrants a name change. RMD Open. 2019;5:e000890.
14. Frighi V, Smith M, Andrews TM, Clifton L, Collins GS, Fuller A, et al. Incidence of fractures in people with intellectual disabilities over the life course: a retrospective matched cohort study. EClinicalMedicine. 2022;52:101656.
15. Jones JT, Kitchen J, Talib N. Down Syndrome-Associated Arthritis (DA): Diagnostic and Management Challenges. Pediatric Health Med Ther. 2022;13:53-62.
16. Juj H, Emery H. The arthropathy of Down syndrome: an underdiagnosed and under-recognized condition. J Pediatr. 2009;154(2):234-8.
17. Kamalakar A, Harris JR, McKelvey KD, Suva LJ. Aneuploidy and skeletal health. Curr Osteoporos Rep. 2014;12(3):376-82.
18. Maranho DA, Fuchs K, Kim YJ, Novais EN. Hip Instability in Patients With Down Syndrome. J Am Acad Orthop Surg. 2018;26(13):455-462. [Erratum in: J Am Acad Orthop Surg. 2018;26(17):625]
19. Mendez AA, Keret D, MacEwen GD. Treatment of patello-femoral instability in Down's syndrome. Clin Orthop Relat Res. 1988;(234):148-58.
20. Merrick J, Ezra E, Josef B, Hendel D, Steinberg DM, Wientroub S. Musculoskeletal problems in Down Syndrome European Paediatric Orthopaedic Society Survey: the Israeli sample. J Pediatr Orthop B. 2000;9(3):185-92.
21. Mik G, Gholve PA, Scher DM, Widmann RF, Green DW. Down syndrome: orthopedic issues. Curr Opin Pediatr. 2008;20(1):30-6.
22. Milbrandt TA, Johnston CE 2nd. Down syndrome and scoliosis: a review of a 50-year experience at one institution. Spine (Phila Pa 1976). 2005;30(18):2051-5.

23. Myśliwiec A, Posłuszny A, Saulicz E, Doroniewicz I, Linek P, Wolny T, et al. Atlanto-axial Instability in People with Down's Syndrome and its Impact on the Ability to Perform Sports Activities - A Review. J Hum Kinet. 2015;48:17-24.
24. Perez EP, Parenti S, Polk J, Jo C, Riccio AI. The Ponseti Method for the Treatment of Clubfeet Associated with Down Syndrome: A Single-institution 18-year Experience. J Pediatr Orthop. 2023;43(2):e106-10.
25. Pueschel SM, Herndon JH, Gelch MM, Senft KE, Scola FH, Goldberg MJ. Symptomatic atlantoaxial subluxation in persons with Down syndrome. J Pediatr Orthop. 1984;4(6): 682-8.
26. Rako K, Ranade S, Allen A. (2021). Orthopaedic Management in Down Syndrome. In J Pediatr Orthop Soc North Am. 2021;3(2):283.
27. Talmac MA, Kadhim M, Rogers KJ, Holmes L Jr, Miller F. Legg-Calvé-Perthes disease in children with Down syndrome. Acta Orthop Traumatol Turc. 2013;47(5):334-8.
28. van Gijzen AFM, Rouers EDM, van Douveren FQMP, Dieleman J, Hendriks JGE, Halbertsma FJJ, et al. Developmental dysplasia of the hip in children with Down syndrome: comparison of clinical and radiological examinations in a local cohort. Eur J Pediatr. 2019;178(4): 559-64.

CHAPTER 10

Hematological Abnormalities in Children with Down Syndrome

Sankar VH

INTRODUCTION

Hematological disorders are among the most common medical complications in patients with Down syndrome (DS). Cancer-based registries suggest that there is 20-fold increased risk of acute lymphoblastic leukemia (ALL) and 150-fold increase risk of acute myeloblastic leukemia in children <5 years. Neonates with DS also have been noted to have higher hemoglobin, nucleated red cells, macrocytosis, target cells, and basophilic stippling. Thrombocytopenia is common; with often giant platelets in circulation. Total lymphocyte count is reduced.

IRON DEFICIENCY/IRON DEFICIENCY ANEMIA

Prevalence of iron deficiency/iron deficiency anemia (ID/IDA) is found to be similar to general population in most of the studies. However, presence of macrocytosis in children with DS may contribute to difficulty in the diagnosis using red cell indices in this group of population. Combination of complete CBC (including red cell distribution width) and serum ferritin, transferrin saturation provides best utility in diagnosing ID/IDA in a child with DS.

For children with DS, current guidelines recommend a complete blood count (CBC) at birth and screening hemoglobin levels in children without any additional risk factors for ID/IDA. If any risk factor of ID/IDA is present or hemoglobin level is <11 g/dL, evaluation of ferritin and CRP is recommended. Transferrin saturation also can be used as an additional measure (if available), which is having the highest sensitivity for ID/IDA.

TRANSIENT LEUKEMIA-DOWN SYNDROME

Transient leukemia of DS (TL-DS) should be defined as the presence of a GATA1 mutation together with a peripheral blood blast percentage >10% and/or clinical features suggestive of TL-DS in a child with DS including mosaic trisomy 21. TL-DS is a preferred terminology for transient abnormal myelopoiesis (TAM) or transient myeloproliferative disorder (TMD) to explain the malignant nature of the condition. TAM/TMD gives a misleading impression of benign nature. About 5–30% of children with DS develop TL.

In around 28% of newborns with DS, hematopoietic cells acquire mutations in gene encoding GATA1, a transcription factor in megakaryocytic-erythroid lineage. This may be clinically silent or result in preleukemia/TMD. It can be observed in all types of DS.

Clinical features can range from asymptomatic to extremely sick babies with jaundice (conjugated hyperbilirubinemia and raised transaminases), skin rash, ascites, hepatosplenomegaly, respiratory distress with pleural effusion, low cardiac output due to pericardial effusion, and hydrops like features. The presence of one or more of the clinical features in the absence of a clear alternative explanation in a neonate with DS should lead to early suspicion and evaluation for TL-DS.

Investigations show leukocytosis with occasional WBC count >100,000/μL, variable thrombocytopenia and megakaryoblasts with prominent nucleoli and cytoplasmic blebbing. Bone marrow examination is not additionally useful since blast cells originate from the fetal liver and the number of blast cells in bone marrow is variable and less prevalent than in peripheral blood. Blast cell immunophenotyping reveals expression of CD34, CD38 and CD117, myeloid markers (CD33 and CD13), platelet glycoproteins (CD41, CD42b, and CD61), erythroid antigen CD235, absent expression of CD56/CD7, and low expression of CD11a. A deranged coagulation profile is observed in 25% patients.

American Academy of Pediatrics recommends evaluation of blood counts and smears at birth to detect neonates with DS who may need early treatment. All neonates with known, or a high suspicion of DS should be examined for features suggestive of TL-DS (organomegaly, cholestasis and hepatopathy, skin rash, and pericardial and pleural effusions). In addition, they should have a full blood count and blood film requested in the first 3 days of life and a formal assessment of the peripheral blood blast cell percentage performed by a hematologist with experience in reviewing neonatal blood films. Babies in whom clinical examination and blast cell percentage indicate that TL-DS is likely should have additional tests considered—liver function tests including conjugated bilirubin if the baby has significant jaundice, chest X-ray, echocardiogram, and abdominal ultrasound. A threshold of >10% peripheral blood blast in the first week of life will detect most cases of TL-DS. Higher the blast cell count is more specific for TL-DS. GATA1 mutation testing is recommended in newborns with 10–20% of blast cells to prevent overdiagnosis. After 1 week, the prevalence may be underestimated since blast cell count will often fall rapidly after birth. Other factors may interfere like falsely low count in severe intrauterine growth restriction (IUGR) babies or in placental insufficiency.

The combination of one or more truncating GATA1 mutation with no increased blast cells percentage in a neonate with DS is termed as silent TL-DS. Rate of transformation of silent TL-DS to myeloid leukemia (ML-DS) is <3% compared to classical TL-DS where the transformation rate is 10–30%. There is currently no evidence of the clinical benefit and cost-effectiveness of routine screening of GATA1 mutation in all children with DS.

Most of the babies with TL-DS (80–90%) will require only observation and monitoring of blood counts. The counts will reduce and the condition will resolve spontaneously by 2–3 months of age. Those with severe symptoms would need clinical treatment as per protocols recommended by multicenter protocols.

The TL-DS blast cells are extremely sensitive to cytarabine in a dose of 10 mg/m^2 or 0.5–1.5 mg/kg either subcutaneously or intravenously by slow infusion twice a day for 7–14 days. Life-threatening symptoms where early treatment should be started are multiorgan failure, white blood cell count >100 × 10^9/L, hepatopathy, massive hepatosplenomegaly, hydrops fetalis (pleural and pericardial effusion), renal failure, and coagulopathy/disseminated intravascular coagulation (DIC). This will definitely reduce the mortality, however, no apparent reduction in the cumulative incidence of ML-DS. Treated children should be closely monitored because of the risks of cytarabine-associated neutropenia and sepsis. Exchange transfusion and leukapheresis may be of use in acute count reduction but should not be considered the definitive treatment.

Most of the cases resolve spontaneously, however, large prospective studies showed an early mortality of 15–23%. The predominant cause of death is progression of hepatic failure, malignant pericardial/pleural effusion, DIC, renal failure, and severe infections. All children with previous TL-DS or silent TL-DS should be monitored for progression to ML-DS with 3 monthly clinical reviews, blood count, and smear until the age of 2 years. Progression is heralded by falling platelet and WBC counts, with dysplastic changes in peripheral smear.

Fetal TL-DS is detected on ultrasound scanning in the third trimester with hepatomegaly and splenomegaly (80%), hydrops fetalis (31%), pericardial effusion (23%), aberrant liquor volume (15%), cardiac abnormalities (12%), fetal ascites (10%) pleural effusion (8%), and peripheral edema (3%). In situations where clinical features on fetal ultrasound scanning suggestive of TL-DS, fetal blood sampling for fetal blood count (FBC), blood film, liver function tests, and GATA1 mutation analysis should be done. A multidisciplinary management by fetal medicine specialist, neonatologist, pediatric hematologists, and obstetrician is likely to increase the chance of a better outcome by timely delivery and postnatal management.

ACUTE MYELOID LEUKEMIA IN DOWN SYNDROME

After the initial clinical resolution with low-dose cytarabine, around 30% of clinical TL-DS will eventually develop acute ML-DS. The mean age of diagnosis of AML in DS is around 2.2 years compared to 6.7 years in those without DS. Progression to ML-DS does not occur after 5 years of age. ML-DS is usually of M7 phenotype (acute megakaryoblastic leukemia—AMKL) and there may be additional cytogenetic abnormalities in bone marrow. Bone marrow histopathological examination in acute AMKL shows replacement with megakaryoblasts (identified by positive platelet peroxidase reaction and immunophenotyping for glycoprotein IIb/IIIa or the von Willibrand factor protein) and reticulin deposition. Cytogenetic abnormalities in DS-AMKL include presence of trisomy involving chromosomes 8 and 1 as well as monosomy 7 whereas absence of the translocation t(1;22) which is seen in non-DS-AKML.

Myeloid/megakaryocytic leukemia in children with DS is a result of series of genetic events. A trisomic background results in oxidative stress which causes to acquire GATA1 mutation leading to TM-DS. The discovery that mutated GATA1 is unable to suppress E2F transcription in fetal liver cells may explain the cellular origin of TMD. Dosage sensitive genes on chromosome 21 such as ERG and ETS2 (ETS proteins) which contribute to megakaryocyte proliferation. Additional acquired mutations to various genes such as *JAK3, FLT3, MPL*, or *TP53* cause subsequent clonal selection and proliferation.

Children are treated on specific protocols for DS and very high cure rates are observed when compared to those with children who do not have DS. The enhanced sensitivity of DS myeloblasts to Ara-C and other chemotherapeutic agents (daunorubicin, melphalan, mitoxantrone, 4-hydroperoxy-cyclophosphamide, vincristine, etoposide, bleomycin, and pirarubicin) is attributed to dosage effect of genes localized to chromosome number 21 including *CBS* gene.

ACUTE LYMPHOBLASTIC LEUKEMIA IN DOWN SYNDROME

The DS-ALL is a unique entity that is characterized by a largely distinct subset of mutations, including trisomy 21, high rates of CRLF2 overexpression, and JAK2 mutations. Children with DS are at a 20-fold increased risk for acute DS-ALL. There are some unique features of ALL in children with DS. These include the predominance of Caucasians, significant rarity of infant ALL and a paucity of T cell ALL (most cases are B-cell phenotype). Moreover, favorable cytogenetics such as ETV6-RUNX1, double trisomy (trisomy of 4 and 10) and high hyperdiploidy, as well as unfavorable cytogenetics such as BCR-ABL1 and MLL rearrangements, are less common in DS-ALL than non-DS ALL.

Standard therapy is generally used for DS-ALL, but the unique toxicity profiles of patients with DS bring challenges. Most of the drugs causes severe complications during induction phase leading to mortality. Overall, the outcome is lower than general pediatric population due to dose reduction of drugs in view of increase toxicity. Although hematopoietic stem cell transplantation (HSCT) remains a viable option for those with high risk or relapsed ALL, the data on HSCT in patients with DS are limited and the role in relapsed patients with DS remains unclear. Novel targeted therapies like chimeric antigen receptor (CAR) T cells appear to be a viable option for DS-ALL.

CONCLUSION

Children with DS are particularly vulnerable to a range of hematological disorders. Iron deficiency anemia is frequently observed and should be actively monitored and managed accordingly. TL-DS (also known as TAM or TMD), unique to neonates with DS, typically resolves spontaneously but requires close surveillance due to its potential progression to ML-DS. Notably, children with DS have a markedly increased risk of both AML and ALL, though with distinct clinical features and treatment responses. These associations underline the importance of vigilant hematological monitoring in DS, as early detection and tailored intervention can significantly impact outcomes.

SUGGESTED READING

1. Hart SJ, Zimmerman K, Linardic CM, Cannon S, Pastore A, Patsiogiannis V, et al. Detection of iron deficiency in children with Down syndrome. Genet Med. 2020;22(2):317-25.
2. John ST, Gayathri K, Ahmed S, Multtani KS, Menon PSN, Kumar RK, et al. Consensus Statement of the Neurodevelopmental Pediatrics Chapter of Indian Academy of Pediatrics (IAP) on the Management of Children With Down Syndrome. Indian Pediatr. 2023;60(4):298-307.
3. Khan I, Malinge S, Crispino J. Myeloid leukemia in Down syndrome. Crit Rev Oncog. 2011;16(1-2):25-36.
4. Lee P, Bhansali R, Izraeli S, Hijiya N, Crispino JD. The biology, pathogenesis and clinical aspects of acute lymphoblastic leukemia in children with Down syndrome. Leukemia. 2016;30(9):1816-23.
5. Tunstall O, Bhatnagar N, James B, Norton A, O'Marcaigh AS, Watts T, et al; British Society for Haematology. Guidelines for the investigation and management of Transient Leukaemia of Down Syndrome. Br J Haematol. 2018;182(2):200-211.
6. Webb D, Roberts I, Vyas P. Haematology of Down syndrome. Arch Dis Child Fetal Neonatal Ed. 2007;92(6):F503-7.

CHAPTER 11

Renal and Urinary Tract Abnormalities

Gayathri K

INTRODUCTION

Renal anomalies in Down syndrome (DS) are considerably higher than in non-DS population. It is approximately 3.5 times higher among live born infants with DS. Children with DS have significantly smaller kidneys and lower number of glomeruli than age-matched controls. There is also evidence of decreased kidney function in these individuals and increased risk of complications.

CAKUT (congenital anomalies of kidney and urinary tract) include a varied group of malformations caused by alterations in the renal embryology. In DS, the CAKUT group include:

- Renal hypoplasia—underdeveloped kidneys with low nephron count
- Renal agenesis—absence of one or both kidneys
- Horseshoe kidney—fusion of lower poles of both kidneys
- Vesicoureteric reflux (VUR)—in which urine flows back from the bladder to the ureter.
- Posterior urethral valve—in males an obstructive membrane in the urethra causes bladder dysfunction and kidney damage.
- Megaureter and hydronephrosis—enlarged ureter due to obstruction or reflux, leading to kidney damage.
- Bladder dysfunction—weak bladder contractions due to neurological impairment leading to urinary retention and infections.
- Epispadias and hypospadias—congenital anomalies of the urethral opening, affecting its position on the penis. In hypospadias, the urethral opening is located on the ventral (underside) of the penis instead of tip. Abnormal fetal androgen levels and associated urogenital anomalies are the possible causes for this. In epispadias, the urethral opening is on the dorsal side of the penis.
- Undescended testes—prevalence of 10–50%. Low testosterone levels and abnormal gonadotrophin signaling impair testicular descent in DS.
- *Renal cysts:* There is substantial increase in the incidence of both micro- and macrocysts. Autosomal recessive polycystic kidney disease is common in children with DS due to its gene located on chromosome 21. These are often asymptomatic unless they are large or compress kidney structures. They indicate underlying kidney disease and require follow-up. There is also higher risk of urinary tract infection (UTI) if they are associated with obstructive anomalies.

GLOMERULAR DISEASES

Glomerular disease usually appears between 2nd and 3rd decade of life. IgA nephropathy and focal segmental glomerular sclerosis are the most frequent pathologies, though minimal change disease and membranous nephropathy have also been reported. It has also been suggested that the immune function associated with DS may predispose children to postinfectious glomerulonephritis. Reduced nephron mass may predispose to glomerular hyperfiltration and injury. Immune dysregulation, genetic factors, metabolic syndrome, and hypertension are also other contributory factors. They require nephrology follow-up for early detection and monitoring. Early screening for proteinuria and kidney function is essential especially in those with congenital kidney anomalies.

Hyperuricemia and hyperuricosuria have also been reported in individuals with DS. Increased purine metabolism, reduced uric acid clearance, oxidative stress, inflammation, dietary, and metabolic factors are the possible causes for the same. Hyperuricemia increases the risk of gout, kidney stones, and chronic kidney disease. Dietary modifications (reducing purine-rich foods, increasing hydration), medications (allopurinol or febuxostat) may be needed to manage this condition.

URODYNAMIC INVOLVEMENT

Children with DS usually attain continence by 4–5 years, which is delayed when compared with other children. However, they can develop secondary urinary incontinence. Urodynamic involvement is seen in up to 30% of children and 8.7% adults with DS. Dysfunctional voiding is common, should be investigated and managed appropriately to prevent long-term renal disease. A non-neurogenic bladder is considered to be related to functional bladder outlet obstruction due to detrusor sphincter dyssynergia. This is considered to be primarily an acquired condition. However, in DS this may be a part of congenital bladder dysfunction, rather than an acquired phenomenon. Hence all children with DS should have a history of bladder function taken.

Urodynamic Findings in Down Syndrome

- Detrusor overactivity—involuntary bladder contractions during filling, leading to urgency, frequency and incontinence. It is due to neurological immaturity.
- Dysfunctional voiding/detrusor-sphincter dyssynergia (DSD)—lack of coordination between bladder contraction and urethral sphincter relaxation, can cause urinary retention, high postvoid residual urine and increased risk of infections.
- Reduced bladder compliance—some individuals with DS have low-compliance bladders, the bladder becomes stiff and does not expand properly. It can lead to high intravesical pressures, can damage the kidneys over time.
- Incomplete emptying and high postvoid residuals—poor bladder contractions or inadequate relaxation of the urinary sphincter can lead to urinary retention and increase the risk of recurrent UTI.
- Nocturnal enuresis and day time incontinence—due to delayed bladder control development, sensory deficits, and hypotonia. It is also due to persistence of infantile voiding patterns.

Management

- *Urodynamic studies:* Bladder pressure testing helps to identify detrusor overactivity, impaired compliance, or dysfunctional voiding.
- *Behavioral and supportive strategies:* Timed voiding and pelvic floor therapy.
- *Pharmacologic therapy:* Anticholinergics (detrusor overactivity) and alpha blockers (dysfunctional voiding).

TESTICULAR TUMORS

In individuals with DS, the lifetime risk of testicular germ cell tumor is 6–50 times higher than in the general population. Undescended testes, chromosomal abnormalities, and hormonal imbalances may be the reason.

Common testicular tumors in DS are:

- *Germ cell tumors*: They are again of two types:
  1. Seminomas—less common in DS, typically occur in adults, slow growing, and good prognosis
  2. Nonseminomatous germ cell tumor—more common in DS, seen in infants and young children
- *Gonadoblastoma*—associated with dysgenetic gonads. It can transform into malignant germ cell tumors.

Regular follow-up is needed for early detection of testicular tumors after the age of 15 years.

RECOMMENDATIONS

- A thorough examination in the newborn period will identify anomalies such as undescended testes, hypospadias, and epispadias.
- After birth, it would be favorable that all patients with DS undergo a renal ultrasound during the first week of life, given the possibility of renal hypoplasia/agenesis or obstructive uropathy, especially when an adequate prenatal USG was not performed.
- If there are symptoms of urinary incontinence or recurrent UTI or VUR or a decrease in estimated glomerular filtration rate is detected, the existence of an associated vesical dysfunction should be considered and a urological evaluation should be done.

CONCLUSION

Since the incidence of renal anomalies are more in DS, a high index of suspicion should be kept in mind, and it should be picked up early to avoid complications. The recommendations noted above would be helpful in this matter.

SUGGESTED READING

1. Hardie C, Puri R. Renal and Urinary Tract Abnormalities. In: Newton RW, Puri S, Marder L (Eds). Down Syndrome Current Perspectives. London: Mac Keith Press; 2015. pp. 181-6.
2. Kute VB, Vanikar AV, Shah PR, Gumber MR, Patel HV, Engineer DP, et al. Down syndrome with end-stage renal disease. Indian J Clin Biochem. 2013;28(4):429-32.
3. Ranchin B, Bidault V, Zekre F, DeMul A, Sanlaville D, Bacchetta J. Kidney and urological involvement in Down syndrome: frequent, underestimated, but associated with impaired quality of life and risk of kidney failure. Pediatr Nephrol. 2024;39(2):347-355.
4. Safdar OY, Albloushy RI, Sait SH, Almadani SH, Ismail AA. Incidence and outcome of renal anomalies in children with down syndrome. AMJ. 2018;11(1):1-5.

CHAPTER 12

Gastrointestinal Manifestations of Down Syndrome

Riyaz Arakkal

INTRODUCTION

Children and adults with Down syndrome (DS) exhibit gastrointestinal symptoms from time to time, such as recurrent vomiting, diarrhea, constipation, and abdominal pain. Most of these usually resolve without any specific treatment. However, some children with DS (about 10%) may develop specific structural and functional disorders of the gastrointestinal system.

STRUCTURAL DISORDERS

The oral manifestations of DS are mouth breathing, scrotal tongue, pseudomacroglossia, delayed teeth eruption, missing and malformed teeth, microdontia, malocclusion, periodontal disease, prolonged retention of primary teeth, supernumerary teeth, diastema, and bruxism. The incidence of dental caries in toddlers is reported to be comparatively low in DS. However, the cause of this is unclear; though it could be due to delayed teeth eruption, differences in saliva composition, and a lower incidence of cariogenic bacteria.

Scrotal tongue or lingua plicata is a benign condition usually seen in DS. It may also be seen in normal children and other rare genetic diseases such as Melkersson-Rosenthal syndrome. It is characterized by the development of deep horizontal fissures on the dorsal and lateral surface of the tongue, similar to the topography of the scrotum. It does not require any specific treatment except for good oral hygiene. The top surface of the tongue should be brushed to remove food debris from the fissures.

In DS, the oropharynx is relatively small, and so there is limited space for the normal-sized tongue to be accommodated in the oral cavity. This causes "pseudomacroglossia/relative macroglossia" **(Fig. 1)**.

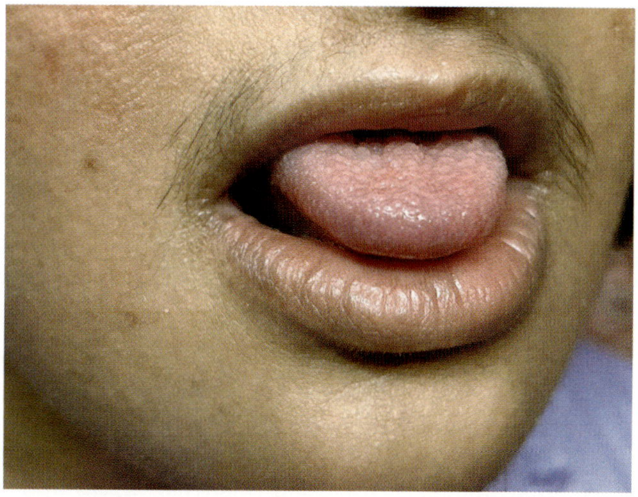

Fig 1: Pseudomacroglossia in Down syndrome (DS).

Drooling of saliva (*sialorrhea*) is a distressing problem in DS. It is due to multiple factors such as intellectual disability, hypotonia of muscles, relative macroglossia, and an open mouth posture. Due to the decrease in the normal control of sensation of the mouth and throat, the child is not able to swallow saliva. In anterior sialorrhea, the excessive saliva spills onto the face and clothes, causing social issues, while in posterior sialorrhea, the child may aspirate saliva into the lungs, resulting in recurrent pneumonia.

These infants are prone to develop gastroesophageal reflux disease (GERD) as they spend more time in the supine position, and muscle tone in the lower esophageal sphincter may be reduced, thus allowing reflux. Infants with DS are usually given more liquid feeds by their mothers, which may aggravate GER, and are at risk of developing aspiration pneumonia. In all children with DS and chronic cough or recurrent pneumonia, GER should be excluded. Many such children are mistakenly treated as having persistent asthma with drugs such as salbutamol, which may actually aggravate GER by relaxing the lower esophageal sphincter.

About 5% of children with DS develop various types of gastrointestinal tract anomalies such as atresias of the esophagus, duodenum, jejunum, and ileum. Malrotation, imperforate anus, Hirschsprung disease, annular pancreas, and Meckel's diverticulum are more common in DS compared to the general population. Others include tracheoesophageal fistula, duodenal web, imperforate anus, omphalocele, etc. The incidence of achalasia cardia is high in children with DS.

The most common gastrointestinal anomaly of DS is duodenal atresia (6%). About 20–30% of children with duodenal atresia have DS **(Fig. 2)**.

In about 80% of neonates with duodenal atresia, the obstruction is beyond the ampulla of Vater. Hence, the neonate presents with persistent bilious vomiting and abdominal distention right from birth onward. Radiograph of abdomen shows the classic "double-bubble" appearance, in which the proximal bubble is due to the distended stomach, and the distal bubble is due to the dilated duodenal bulb. This radiologic sign is diagnostic of duodenal atresia, and other investigations are usually not required. Some children with DS who have incomplete obstruction due to fenestrated duodenal membranes may present later in life with recurrent vomiting. Annular pancreas, first described in 1818 by Tiedemann, is the most common congenital anomaly of the pancreas in children. It is associated with other congenital anomalies, especially duodenal atresia, and is also common in DS. Double-bubble appearance may also be seen in annular pancreas. Recent studies have shown that the annular pancreas associated with DS may be due to disruptions in hedgehog signaling.

Another important cause of bilious vomiting and abdominal distention in DS is malrotation. Such anomalies of the GI tract may be detected in the antenatal period itself by appropriate imaging techniques so that surgery may be undertaken as early as possible after birth. Almost 50% of neonates with imperforate anus and 10% of children with Hirschsprung have associated DS.

10% of neonates with DS may also have Hirschsprung disease, especially the short segment type, and recent evidence suggests that Down syndrome cell adhesion molecule (DSCAM) on chromosome 21, which belongs to the immunoglobulin superfamily, is a susceptibility locus for Hirschsprung disease **(Figs. 3A and B)**. The usual symptoms are delayed passage of meconium, distended abdomen, poor weight gain, vomiting, and constipation. Associated hypothyroidism may also cause delayed passage of meconium in DS.

Very rarely, some infants with DS may have a dual pathology—both duodenal atresia and Hirschsprung disease. This may cause diagnostic issues as the clinical features of duodenal atresia may overshadow those of Hirschsprung disease. Meckel's diverticulum, the most common congenital malformation within the gastro-intestinal tract, may also be seen in DS.

The prognosis of infants with DS and major anomalies such as duodenal atresia or Hirschsprung disease is usually as good as that of chromosomally normal infants. However, if the infant has additional major anomalies such as congenital heart disease, the mortality may be higher.

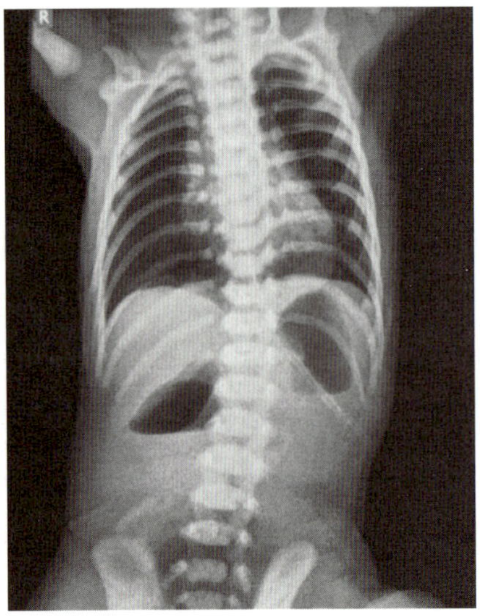

Fig 2: Double bubble in duodenal atresia.
Photo Courtesy: Dr Kesavan T.

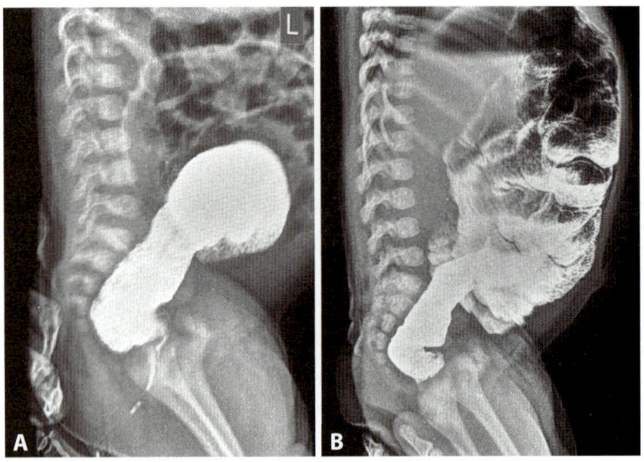

Figs. 3A and B: Barium enema of a child with Hirschsprung disease
Photo Courtesy: Dr VK Gopi.

FUNCTIONAL DISORDERS

In addition to these organic conditions, there is also a high incidence of functional gastrointestinal disorders such as functional constipation, irritable bowel syndrome, and functional dyspepsia in children with DS.

An older child presenting with chronic constipation is a common problem in DS, even in the absence of Hirschsprung disease. Hypotonia, relative inactivity, faulty toilet training and a diet poor in fibers, fruits, and vegetables may all contribute to chronic constipation. Normal meconium history and normal stools till about 1 year help to rule out Hirschsprung disease. These children develop anal fissure due to the passage of very hard stools, resulting in dyschezia, hematochezia, fecal impaction, and encopresis. Rectal examination will show a loaded rectum. Hypothyroidism should always be excluded in such children as it is an important cause of constipation and is common in DS. Intake of a sufficient quantity of fruits and vegetables should be encouraged. The drug of choice is polyethylene glycol, which should be continued till the fissure heals, and the child is able to pass painless type 4 or 5 Bristol stools.

AUTOIMMUNE DISORDERS

Autoimmune diseases such as autoimmune adrenalitis, pernicious anemia, Hashimoto disease, and diabetes mellitus are common in DS. Autoimmune hepatitis may also rarely occur.

Children with DS have a 5- to 16-fold increased risk of developing celiac disease compared with the general population. In view of this strong association, it may be useful to screen children with DS for celiac disease with tissue transglutaminase antibody beginning at 3 years of age and repeated every 2–3 years. These children may present with small bowel diarrhea, failure to thrive, abdominal distension, or constipation. The presence of calcium deficiency, iron deficiency anemia, and elevated transaminases also suggest the possibility of underlying celiac disease in these children. The diagnosis may be confirmed by a positive tissue transglutaminase antibody and small bowel biopsy, and the child should be put on a lifelong gluten-free diet.

DOWN SYNDROME AND LIVER DISEASES

Children with DS are immunocompromised. Hence, the risk of becoming HBsAg carriers is high following exposure to the hepatitis B virus, which is especially true of institutionalized patients with DS. This underscores the importance of hepatitis B vaccination in these children, starting right from birth. Timely vaccination may help to reduce the high incidence of hepatitis A and B infection in DS.

Neonatal cholestasis has been reported in DS, which may be due to the paucity of intrahepatic bile ducts. Biliary atresia per se appears to be rare in DS.

As per a study from Brazil, in children with DS <3 years, 9% had either gallstones or biliary sludge. Hence, children with DS who are at risk of developing cholelithiasis and biliary sludge should be monitored throughout the neonatal period with serial ultrasound scans. Drugs that may precipitate biliary sludge, such as ceftriaxone, should be avoided in these children. They may require cholecystectomy if they develop cholecystitis.

CONCLUSION

Gastrointestinal malformations may be seen in about 5% of children with DS. Some of these are life threatening, like duodenal atresia and malrotation, and should be ruled out in any neonate with bilious vomiting and abdominal distention. Delayed passage of meconium and abdominal distension suggest Hirschsprung disease. GERD, which is also common, may be mistaken for asthma and treated with drugs that decrease lower esophageal sphincter pressure, such as salbutamol, thereby aggravating reflux. Functional constipation, which is more common in older children with DS, should be treated with polyethylene glycol, toilet training, and other supportive measures. Hypothyroidism should always be ruled out in such children.

SUGGESTED READING

1. Amiel J, Sproat-Emison E, Garcia-Barcelo M, Lantieri F, Burzynski G, Borrego S, et al. Hirschsprung disease, associated syndromes and genetics: A review. J Med Genet. 2008;45:1-14.
2. Amil Dias J, Walker-Smith J. Down's syndrome and coeliac disease. J Pediatr Gastroenterol Nutr. 1990;10:41-3.
3. Boëchat MC, Silva KS, Llerena JC Jr, Boëchat PR. Cholelithiasis and biliary sludge in Down's syndrome patients. Sao Paulo Med J. 2007;125:329-32.
4. Chang CH, Kim JH, Lee SJ, Lee DS, Kim DK, Choi SM, et al. A case of Nonsyndromic paucity of interlobular bile ducts in Down syndrome. J Korean Pediatr Soc. 1999;42:858-62.
5. de Bortoli N, Martinucci I, Savarino E, Bellini M, Bredenoord AJ, Franchi R, et al. Proton pump inhibitor responders who are not confirmed as GERD patients with impedance and pH monitoring: who are they? Neurogastroenterol Motil. 2014;26:28-35.

6. Eksarko P, Nazir S, Kessler E, LeBlanc P, Zeidman M, Asarian AP, et al. Duodenal web associated with malrotation and review of literature. J Surg Case Rep. 2013;2013(12):rjt110.
7. Ibrahim ATA, Hamdy AM, Elhodhod MA. Prevalence of functional gastrointestinal disorders among school-aged children and adolescents, a multicenter study. QJM: An International Journal of Medicine. 2020;113(Suppl 1): hcaa063-029.
8. Jannot AS, Pelet A, Henrion-Caude A, Chaoui A, Masse-Morel M, Arnold S, et al. Chromosome 21 scan in Down syndrome reveals DSCAM as a predisposing locus in Hirschsprung's disease. PLoS ONE. 2013;8(5):e62519.
9. Lainakis N, Antypas S, Panagidis A, Alexandrou I, Kambouri K, Kyriazis C, et al. Annular pancreas in two consecutive siblings: an extremely rare case. Eur J Pediatr Surg. 2005;15:364-8.
10. Puri P, Guiney EJ. Intrahepatic biliary atresia in Down's syndrome. J Pediatr Surg. 1975;10:423-4.
11. Stoll C, Alembik Y, Dott B, Roth MP. Study of Down syndrome in 238,942 consecutive births. Ann Genet. 1998;41(1):44-51.

CHAPTER 13

Dermatological Manifestations in Down Syndrome

Abhay Mani Martin

INTRODUCTION

Trisomy 21 or Down syndrome (DS) has protean manifestations on the skin and can be seen on the skin, hair, and appendageal organs. Lesions on the skin can be an early contributory marker to detect trisomy 21. Some lesions are seen at birth, and some lesions evolve as the child grows into adolescence and adulthood. The skin lesions in this syndrome were noted earliest by Seguin (1846). The skin in early childhood is soft and velvety. It later turns dry or xerotic as the child advances into late childhood. There is no formal classification of skin disorders in trisomy 21, and hence, the manifestations are listed as below, depending on the area of involvement.

HAIR ANOMALIES

Newborns with DS typically have normal hair at birth, which tends to become finer and hypopigmented as they grow older. Alopecia areata, characterized by focal areas of hair loss, is a common association with trisomy 21 (**Figs. 1A and B**). Defects in T-cell function as well as immunoglobulin G (IgG) deficiencies are the attributable factors. It is more severe, recurrent, and more resistant to treatment.

ORAL LESIONS

Persons with trisomy 21 have macroglossia with a fissured tongue. This, along with hypertrophied papillae on the tongue, geographic tongue, cheilitis, and angular cheilitis were prominent findings in an Iranian study of 100 patients with DS.

The incidence of fissured or scrotal tongue is as high as 80% in DS compared to 5% in the general population. Geographic tongue is another common lingual anomaly and is characterized by superficial eroded areas on the tongue in patches.

Cheilitis is a common occurrence in this population and is attributable to multiple factors including repetitive trauma, candidal infections, angular cheilitis of

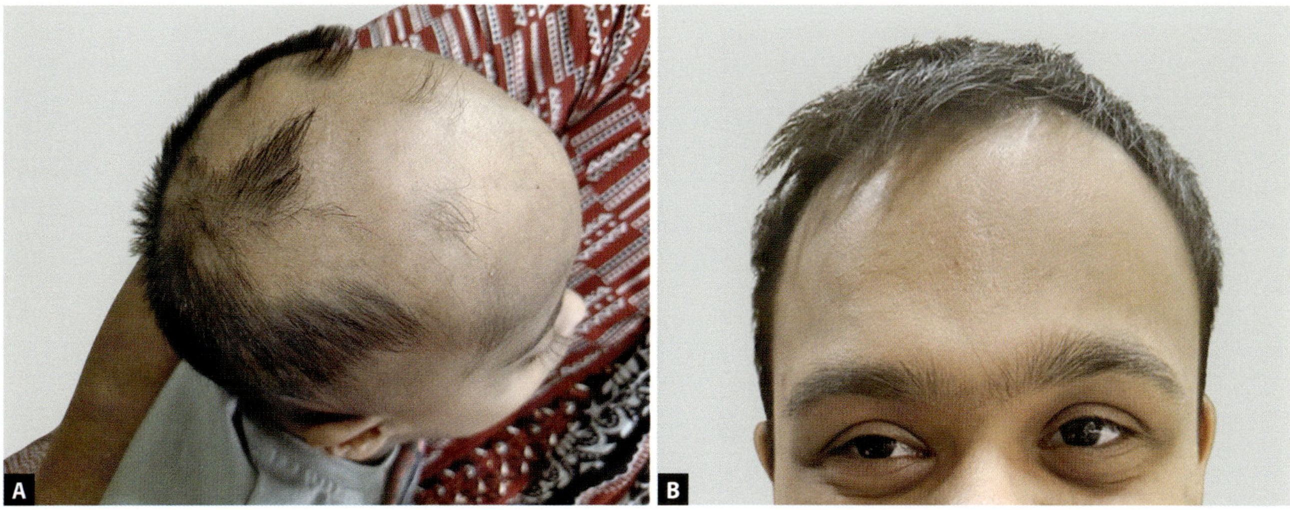

Figs. 1A and B: (A) Alopecia areata—a common hair association in trisomy 21; (B) Alopecia areata.

avitaminosis, and actinic cheilitis. Atopy in these patients also predisposes to cheilitis.

Periodontitis is yet another common association in trisomy 21 with no specific identifiable etiopathogenetic factor for predisposition. Decreased salivation, microbial colonization, impaired immune mechanisms including neutrophil and innate immune deficiencies, capillary and microvascular fragility, disordered connective tissue, and abnormal teeth alignment have all been implicated. The incidence is very high in patients <30 years of age and can lead to horizontal bone loss in the lower anteriors.

DERMATOGLYPHICS

Single palmar crease, also called Simian crease (Mongolian crease in early literature), is considered a hallmark of trisomy 21 (incidence of 40–50%). This should serve as an early marker in infancy to detect and plan strategies for further management of such babies. Children with trisomy 21 have a high incidence of loops and a low incidence of whorls. The most common digital pattern is 10 ulnar loops in the hypothenar eminence of the palms. A radial loop on the fifth finger occurs in 4% of children with trisomy 21 and in only 0.3% of control subjects. An arched tibial (At) pattern in the hallucal area of soles occurs more frequently in patients with DS (50%) as against controls (0.3%).

SKIN FINDINGS

Signs of premature skin aging such as skin atrophy, lentigines, xerosis, and canities are more often noted in persons with DS **(Fig. 2)**.

Eczemas are often noted and may present in their acute form with oozing, vesiculation, and crusting or in a chronic form as lichenification. Frequent skin barrier breakdown, leading to secondary bacterial infections and impetiginization, is common. Recurrences of eczema are very common and are attributable to repetitive trauma by itching. Eczemas occur in children with DS secondary to ichthyosis, asteatosis, seborrheic dermatitis, or atopic dermatitis.

Psoriasis as an association with DS has not been studied in detail. Obesity is a risk factor for psoriasis in association with DS **(Fig. 3)**. However, there are occasional case reports of association of psoriasis and cardiac disease risk, including myocardial infarction, palmoplantar psoriasis, and psoriatic arthritis. Success in the treatment of psoriasis with biologics (such as adalimumab and etanercept) and Janus kinase (JAK) inhibitors (such as tofacitinib) has been variable. TNF alpha inhibitors such as etanercept have shown failures in patients with DS and psoriasis.

INFECTIONS

Persons with DS are more prone to infections—bacterial, fungal, and parasitic. Folliculitis, furuncles, cellulitis, and impetiginized wounds are a common occurrence, either de novo or as a part of the atopic dermatitis spectrum.

Fungal infections, including candidiasis in flexural areas due to obesity, angular cheilitis, and dermatophytic infections such as tinea pedis and tinea corporis, are common. Pityrosporum folliculitis presents as multiple small follicular and perifollicular papular eruptions on the intermammary and interscapular regions.

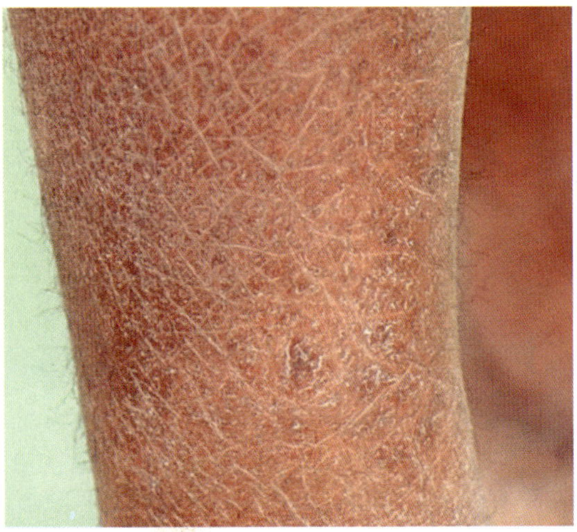

Fig. 2: Xerosis of skin and skin atrophy due to rapid skin aging.

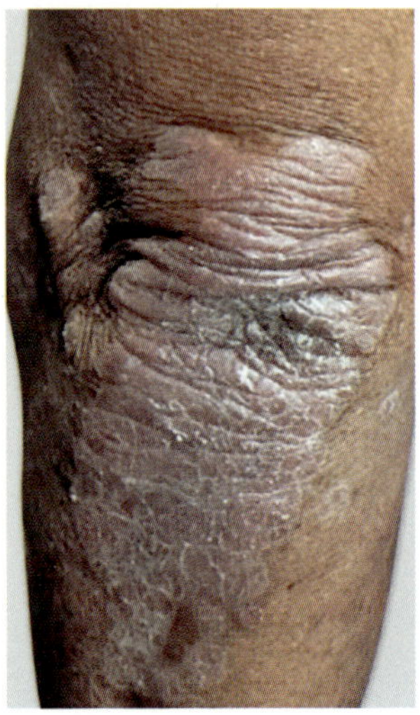

Fig. 3: Psoriasis as an association with trisomy 21.

Ectoparasitic and endoparasitic infections are known associations. Crusted scabies, a more severe form of scabies characterized by thick scaly crusted lesions on the interdigital web spaces, elbows, and buttocks, is more common in this population. It is presumed to be due to a lower immune response to colonization of these mites as well as due to poor hygiene in some community living units.

ASSOCIATED CONDITIONS

Persons with DS have a higher incidence of immune-mediated illnesses such as alopecia areata and vitiligo. Seborrheic dermatitis, palmoplantar hyperkeratosis, keratosis pilaris, and premature graying are some of the other prominent findings recorded in the literature. Other rarer associations include calcinosis cutis, milia, syringomas, hidradenitis suppurativa **(Fig. 4)**, and unusual forms of elastosis perforans serpiginosa (EPS).

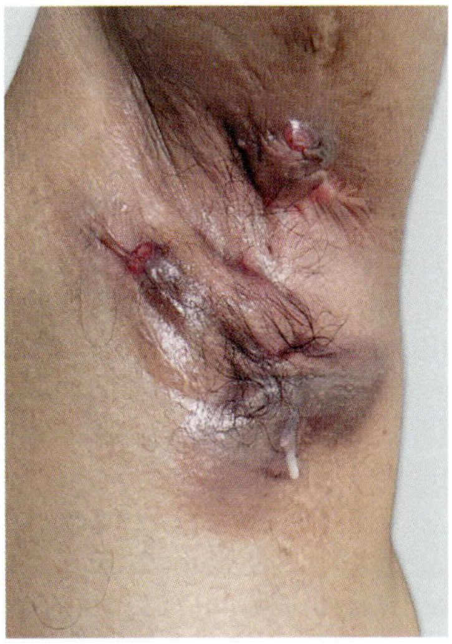

Fig. 4: Hidradenitis suppurativa.

Vascular anomalies such as cutis marmorata, characterized by a reticulate pattern of vascular network, and acrocyanosis are common and are attributable to poor peripheral circulation. Vascular anomalies may also be seen secondary to the effects of congenital heart disease, which is common with DS.

Skin manifestations of hematologic conditions such as leukemia and myelodysplastic syndrome, which are noted more in DS, may manifest as vesiculopustules, papular, and nodular eruptions.

CONCLUSION

Trisomy 21 has myriad manifestations which serve not only as cutaneous markers of recognizing the disease but also markers of underlying disease associations such as autoimmune disorders, infections, or malignancy. A keen eye to elicit the cutaneous symptoms and signs may help in early recognition and intervention.

SUGGESTED READING

1. Dominguez-Cruz JJ, Delgado B. Dermatological Manifestations of Down Syndrome. Genetics and Etiology of Down Syndrome. InTech; 2011. Available from: http://dx.doi.org/10.5772/19321.
2. Lam M, Lu JD, Elhadad L, Sibbald C, Alhusayen R. Common Dermatologic Disorders in Down Syndrome: Systematic Review. JMIR Dermatol. 2022;5(1):e33391.
3. Madan V, Williams J, Lear JT. Dermatological manifestations of Down's syndrome. Clin Exp Dermatol. 2006;31(5):623-9.
4. Ryan C, Vellody K, Belazarian L, Rork JF. Dermatologic conditions in Down syndrome. Pediatr Dermatol. 2021;38(Suppl 2):49-57.
5. Sureshbabu R, Kumari R, Ranugha S, Sathyamoorthy R, Udayashankar C, Oudeacoumar P. Phenotypic and dermatological manifestations in Down Syndrome. Dermatol Online J. 2011;17(2).

CHAPTER 14

Dental Care in Persons with Down Syndrome

Nidhi Gupta, Anurag Gupta

INTRODUCTION

People with Down syndrome (DS) or trisomy 21 present with significant oral and dental health-related challenges and are considered to be at twice at risk for dental diseases compared to their peers. Anatomical and developmental irregularities in the middle third of the face often result in impaired functions such as chewing, swallowing, and speech.

People with DS may have varied dental needs, but the most common underlying feature is neglect of dental problems. While the caregivers are already grappling with other health issues, dental problems are mostly neglected or delayed for later.

On the other hand, providing dental treatment to persons with DS is not an easy task for dental professionals because of poor cooperation from the patients and poor compliance with instructions that are given. Many a time, people with intellectual disabilities can be very noncompliant and sometimes aggressive in the dental chair, thereby making dental procedures impossible to be carried out.

It is known that oral hygiene plays a vital role in overall wellbeing. Dental care given early to children with DS is beneficial in many ways. Timely and regular consultation with a dentist can benefit the caregiver by providing them with adequate knowledge and equip them in creating a "dental home" whose benefits can go a long way.

COMMON ORAL PROBLEMS IN DOWN SYNDROME

Common oral problems can be categorized broadly into two categories:

1. Hard tissues-related, i.e., teeth and jaw bones
2. Soft tissues-related, i.e., tongue, gums, cheeks, and lips

Hard Tissues-related

Delayed Eruption/Noneruption of Teeth

It is commonly found that the child with DS may show delayed eruption of baby teeth. This means that while a non-DS child may show teeth appearance as early as 6 months and complete the eruption of all milk teeth by 24–30 months of age, a child with DS may start teething late, and complete eruption may take up to 3 years or 4 years of age. So, it is important that parents and caregivers be aware of this and do not panic unnecessarily.

Hypodontia and Dental Agenesis: Nonformation of Teeth/Congenitally Missing Teeth

A child with DS may exhibit nonformation/congenitally missing baby tooth or teeth, which means that they are not formed by birth, and the tooth buds are absent altogether. In such cases, one or more teeth may be missing. This means that the child will have fewer than 20 milk teeth. Again, there is no need to panic in such cases, but we should strive to keep the remaining ones healthy. To find out about congenitally missing teeth, one will need to take an orthopantomogram X-ray (full mouth—OPG X-ray). It is recommended that such an OPG X-ray be taken by around 4 years of age.

Microdontia: Short Roots/Short Crowns

It is very common to see that the size of teeth, both crown size and root size, is generally smaller in individuals with DS. This is more common in permanent dentition than in primary dentition.

Abnormal Crown and Root Morphology

Enamel hypoplasia and hypocalcification, which may affect both primary and permanent dentitions, are common in DS. This means that the quality of enamel and dentine material in the teeth is not very good and is susceptible to faster wear and tear. Peg-shaped lateral incisor is a very common example.

Spacings

Due to a smaller number of teeth formed or erupted, spacing between the teeth is quite common in individuals with DS.

Over-retained Deciduous Teeth

It is commonly seen in individuals with DS that the milk teeth do not fall out as per schedule. Delay in exfoliation of primary teeth is a relatively common feature here, and this may lead to delayed eruption of permanent teeth or deflection in the path of eruption of permanent teeth.

Double Row Dentition

When the primary teeth do not fall out as per schedule, the permanent teeth may erupt behind and form a second row of teeth. Some parents may find it scary and may panic. But there is nothing to worry about as remedy is available.

V-shaped Upper Jaw/Narrow Upper Jaw

This is a very common feature in individuals with DS and basically indicates the deficient development of the upper jaw (maxilla). The maxilla is not only underdeveloped in width but also in vertical development.

Deep Palate

Deep palate/stair palate/shelf-like palate means that the palatal vault is very steep and is again an indicator of underdevelopment of the maxilla in width.

Crowded Upper Jaw

Since the upper jaw is underdeveloped, it also has inadequate space to accommodate all the teeth in a proper line, thereby leading to crowding of upper teeth.

Dental Crossbite in Front and Side Segment

The maxilla is usually narrower than the mandible, thereby creating a mismatch. This relationship is called a class III type relation and can range from a mild problem wherein only one tooth or a few teeth are in crossbite (reverse relationship) to severe dental crossbite wherein all the teeth are in reverse relationship.

Skeletal Crossbite Ranging from Mild to Severe to Complete Scissors Bite

Since the growth of the maxilla is usually less than the mandible, there is a common tendency for individuals with DS to develop a true skeletal Cl III relationship that manifests a dental crossbite. Again, the severity of the skeletal mal-relationship may range from mild to severe. Proper facial X-rays and evaluation by an orthodontist will be needed to diagnose the exact cause of the Cl III relationship.

Fortunately, now the treatment of such conditions is available even at later ages, and more and more parents come forward to get their wards treated.

Soft Tissues-related

Gingivitis with or without Periodontitis (Gum Disease)

Gingivitis, ranging from moderate to severe forms, with or without periodontitis, acute necrotizing forms, and advanced chronic periodontitis, leading to gingival recession and alveolar bone loss, are quite prevalent in individuals with DS compared to the normal population.

Large Tongue

Children with DS may have a large tongue, or they may have an average-size tongue and a small upper jaw that makes their tongue too large for their mouth.

Fissure Tongue

It is a relatively common feature in persons with DS to find grooves on the top surface of the tongue. While this usually does not present with any problems, very deep grooves may lead to the accumulation of food particles and may be difficult to clean.

Geographic Tongue

This means that the top surface of the tongue has certain areas which do not have the normal papillae and are of a different color. This leads to the appearance of a map drawn on the tongue. This condition is also called benign migratory glossitis and is not restricted to DS. Usually, it is asymptomatic, but sometimes there may be a loss of certain taste sensations.

Everted and Thick Lower Lip

Due to poor tonicity in the oral region, the lower lip may be hanging loose and everted.

Cracked/Chaffed Lips

The poor tonicity of lip muscles, along with mouth breathing, leads to an absent lip seal, and the lips become dry and chaffed.

Tongue Thrust

The tongue size may be large, and there may be a low sensory ability in the oral cavity, which may lead to the tongue being positioned outward. This makes their tongue to stay out.

Open Mouth Condition

This could be due to a lot of reasons:

- Relatively large tongue, due to which the mouth is constantly open
- Weak and flaccid lip and cheek muscles
- Narrow nasal passages
- Enlarged adenoids and tonsils
- Overall poor sensitivity and perception in the orofacial region

Angular Cheilitis

This essentially means that there is a lesion at the corner of the mouth. This usually occurs as a result of the open mouth and drooling of saliva. There may also be associated vitamin deficiencies.

Mouth Ulcers

Individuals with DS are prone to mouth ulcers, which may be because of many reasons, including thin mucosal oral lining, poor gum health, poor gastrointestinal health, etc.

IMPORTANCE OF DENTAL CARE IN PERSONS WITH DOWN SYNDROME

The oral cavity, with all its soft and hard tissues, serves as a gateway to general, psychological, and social wellbeing. The importance of keeping good oral health has now been emphasized by several researches and publications. But when it comes to the oral health of individuals with DS, it tends to be overlooked.

It is well known that people with DS do not express their problems, or they may not desire a fabulous smile like a neurotypical individual. But they will simply stop chewing or may start showing abnormal or aggressive behavior if there is tooth pain.

Normal oral functions are affected in children with DS right from infancy. This means that either children with DS do not learn these oral functions effectively, or they learn them quite later when compared to typical children. Oral functions that need to be focused in children with DS include chewing, spitting, blowing and holding air in mouth, sucking, and rinsing.

This is primarily because of the reduced sensations in the oral and facial region, as well as low muscle tone. This leads to muscle flaccidity and loose hanging tongue, lips, and cheeks, and an open mouth as mentioned earlier. This low muscle tone greatly affects the development of simple and normal oral functions that are seen, so naturally, in children without DS.

An informed dentist can teach the parents at a very early stage about not just preventive dentistry but also oromotor functional development. It is an established fact that the development and function of oral muscles such as tongue, lips, and cheek have a very significant role in the normal healthy maintenance of teeth and gums. Establishing normal oral function early has additional benefits from an occupational therapy and speech therapy point of view.

Later, deficient jaw development and/or malocclusion of teeth may result in many teens and adults stopping eating normal hard food items such as rotis, and just restricting to a soft diet. Such issues can be tackled if managed early.

Regular dental checkups, dental prophylaxis (cleaning), and preventive dental treatment help in maintaining a healthy oral environment and functionality. And now, with improving technology and inclusive lifestyles, they may also be given better and beautiful smiles.

MANAGEMENT OF PATIENTS WITH DOWN SYNDROME IN A CLINICAL SETTING

Children with DS are usually friendly, but fear of the unknown, with fear of pain/injection, deters them from cooperating for a meaningful examination and procedure. These children usually take more time and sometimes a greater number of visits to become comfortable in a dental setting, and therefore it is very important that the dentist and the staff should be able to give enough time to the child, and that too cheerfully and patiently. It is important to address issues from their point of view and make them as comfortable as possible. The preparation should start from home.

The parents can be asked to resort to the following:

- *Behavior modeling:* If a sibling/cousin is available, then the same can be asked to show good behavior in the dental chair, which the other child can see and copy.
- *Social stories:* Parents should make up social stories around dental treatment before the visit.
- *Dental apps:* There are many apps available on the Google Play Store and Apple Play Store that can be downloaded and used to create a positive mindset regarding dentistry.

Sedation Techniques

Conscious Sedation Techniques

Dentists nowadays use nitrous oxide sedation and other conscious sedation techniques to reduce the anxiety of the patient and perform dental procedures in the dental chair itself. Conscious sedation procedures involving nitrous oxide or IV sedation are generally safe. However, it is always better to have an anesthesiologist present to administer these sedations. Also, the clinic should be equipped with proper equipment to manage the patient in case of an emergency.

Dental Procedures Under General Anesthesia

If the individual, whether a child or an adult with DS, is completely uncooperative on a dental chair, then performing the procedure under general anesthesia (GA) is the only option left. It is now a safe and commonly practiced treatment option, but proper preanesthetic evaluation is mandatory.

Important Points to be Kept in Mind before any Dental Procedure is Done Under General Anesthesia

When the child is scheduled for a procedure under GA, the following should be kept in mind:

- Main treatment should be completed in the same sitting.
- Preventive pit and fissure sealant/varnish treatment for other teeth as well should be done for the prevention of dental carries.
- Any other near-future extraction may also be performed.
- All teeth to be thoroughly assessed for any dental filling/space maintainer/capping, etc.
- If any dental X-rays are pending, then they must be made at the same time.
- Detailed planning for all teeth in the mouth should be done so that the need for a repeat GA in the near future may be avoided.

ADVANCED DENTAL TECHNOLOGY—BOON FOR PERSONS WITH SPECIAL NEEDS

Technology is making life easier in all walks of life. And dentistry is also getting its fair share of technological advancements. Technology can be especially beneficial for persons with special needs, regardless of the disability/special need, whether intellectual or physical. Most of the below-mentioned technologies can be used not only in DS but also in autism, Attention deficit hyperactivity disorder (ADHD), cerebral palsy, and spinal muscular atrophy (SMA).

Anticavity Paints—Pit and Fissure Sealants

These seal the grooves on the chewing surface of the teeth and prevent the ingress of food particles and microbes into these susceptible areas, thereby preventing cavity formation. These have been there in dentistry for a long time but used restrictively in pediatric cases only. They can be used in teens and adults with DS, also with good results.

Orthodontic Treatment for Alignment of Teeth

Modern orthodontic treatment is now more comfortable and less dependent on patient compliance, thereby making it more acceptable and successful.

Dental Aligners such as Invisalign, SureSmile, and Clear Correct

Wireless braces systems called dental aligners are more comfortable, less risky to trauma, and more acceptable.

Digitally Printed Miniscrew or Microimplant-assisted Rapid Palatal Expansion

Palatal expansion was earlier successful only before 11–12 years of age. But now digitally printed *miniscrew or microimplant-assisted rapid palatal expansion (MARPE)* can be done even in later age with good results. MARPE devices are used to achieve a skeletal expansion of the palate and to increase the arch perimeter. This technology really brings much hope for persons with DS, because many parents miss out on getting proper orthodontic advice during the early teen period of their children.

3D Scanning

3D scanning of the teeth and jaws with or without cone beam computed tomography (CBCT) is an excellent tool for treatment planning, record keeping, and long-term comparison. This can also help in 3D printing of appliances apart from the visualization and counseling of parents and families.

AWARENESS AMONG PEDIATRICIANS AND THERAPISTS

Children with DS are regularly seen by pediatricians, speech therapists, occupational therapists, ear, nose, and throat (ENT) specialists, and others, but used to be infrequently seen by a dentist. It is commonly seen that many doctors are not aware of the dental issues, their treatment, and their impact on the life of that person. Many times, the cause of certain behaviors can be traced to an underlying dental problem. In fact, it is possible for therapists and dentists to work hand in hand in developing functional skills in a child with DS.

REFERRAL TO DENTIST—WHY AND WHEN?

Referring a person with DS to a dentist should be done at the appropriate time because every person, whatever the age, will have some dental challenge, big or small. And they do not express it until the problem becomes really big, and a serious intervention such as extraction is all that can be done. People caring for children with DS should update the parents and refer the children at the appropriate time for the needed dental care.

CONCLUSION

The conclusions are detailed in **Flowcharts 1 and 2**. The reference for the chart is included in suggested reading.

SUGGESTED READING

1. Asokan S, Muthu MS, Sivakumar N. Dental caries prevalence and treatment needs of Down syndrome children in Chennai, India. Indian J Dent Res. 2008;19(3):224-9.
2. Bower C, Leonard H, Petterson B. Intellectual disability in Western Australia. J Paediatr Child Health. 2000;36(3): 213-5.
3. Cheng RH, Yiu CK, Leung WK. (2011). Oral Health in Individuals with Down Syndrome. [online] Available from https://www.researchgate.net/publication/221914618_Oral_Health_in_Individuals_with_Down_Syndrome [Last accessed April 2025].
4. Descamps I, Marks LA. Oral health in children with Down syndrome: Parents' views on dental care in Flanders (Belgium). Eur J Paediatr Dent. 2015;16(2):143-8.
5. Goud EVSS, Gulati S, Agrawal A, Pani P, Nishant K, Pattnaik SJ, et al. Implications of Down's syndrome on oral health status in patients: A prevalence-based study. J Family Med Prim Care. 2021;10(11):4247-52.
6. Holt K, Barzel R, Bertness J. Oral Health for Children and Adolescents with Special Health Care Needs: Challenges and Opportunities, 2nd edition. Washington, DC: National Maternal and Child Oral Health Resource Center; 2014.
7. Kanagaraj PP, Gurenlian JR. Oral health considerations for patients with Down syndrome. Decisions Dent. 2021;7: 40-3.
8. Manikandan K, Seshadri S. Down Syndrome Screening in India: Are We There Yet? J Obstet Gynaecol India. 2017; 67(6):393-9.
9. Martins M, Mascarenhas P, Evangelista JG, Barahona I, Tavares V. The Incidence of Dental Caries in Children with Down Syndrome: A Systematic Review and Meta-Analysis. Dent J (Basel). 2022;10(11):205.
10. Oredugba FA. Oral health condition and treatment needs of a group of Nigerian individuals with Down syndrome. Downs Syndr Res Pract. 2007;12(1):72-6.
11. Practical Oral care for people with Down syndrome, National Institute of Dental and Craniofacial Research. US Department of Health and Human Services. https://www.nidcr.nih.gov/sites/default/files/2020-10/practical-oral-care-down-syndrome.pdf.
12. Scalioni F, Carrada CF, Abreu L, Ribeiro RA, Paiva SM. Perception of parents/caregivers on the oral health of children/adolescents with Down syndrome. Spec Care Dentist. 2018;38(6):382-90.

Flowchart 1: For parents regarding importance of dental care in children and adults with Down syndrome.

Basic oral hygiene

Need to keep hard and soft tissues of oral cavity (teeth, gums, tongue, palate) clean and healthy

↓

Prevention of orofacial dysfunction

Not just prevention of oral dysfunction but also establishing proper oral function

↓

Prevention and correction of teeth misalignment in children and teens

Misalingment of teeth and jaws is universal and present in nearly every child with DS. Prevention with early intervention appliances and later correction with orthodontics

↓

Cosmetic dentistry for improving smile of adults

Improved facial look helps in easy acceptance and inclusion in society as more DS adults are getting independent and working

Flowchart 2: Various age-related issues faced by persons with Down syndrome.

Age-related dental care in persons with trisomy 21

Pediatricians/Medical doctors/ Therapists must refer to dentists

For following issues

Infancy 0–1 years
- Counseling on feeding and suckling
- Congenital anomalies such as tongue tie, lip tie, neonatal teeth, and clefts
- Weaning from bottle feeding
- Care for gum pads

1–5 years
- Oromotor therapy – Why, how, when?
- Establishing oral functions such as spitting, sucking, blowing, holding breath, chewing
- Teeth brushing – when, how to start?
- Preventing/treating teeth cavities/decay
- Tongue thrusting, teeth grinding
- Expansion of narrow palate

5–8 years
- Tongue thrusting, drooling, mouth breathing, teeth grinding
- Reinforcing/starting oromotor therapy
- Appliance therapy for palatal expansion, tongue thrusting
- Preventing/treating dental decay
- Reinforcing teeth brushing

8–12 years
- Tongue thrusting, drooling, mouth breathing, teeth grinding
- Preventing/treating dental decay/gum care
- Reinforcing teeth brushing/home care
- Appliance therapy for palatal expansion, tongue thrusting
- Orthodontic treatment for misaligned teeth

Teens
- Tongue thrusting, drooling, mouth breathing, teeth grinding, chewing issues
- Orthodontic treatment for misaligned teeth
- Preventing/treating dental decay
- Reinforcing teeth brushing/home care

Young adults
- Teeth grinding, chewing issues
- Limited orthodontic treatment
- Orthognathic surgery for severe jaw dysplasia
- Preventing/treating dental decay and gum care
- Reinforcing teeth brushing/home care
- Restorative dentistry for missing teeth/decayed teeth
- Cosmetic dentistry for smile improvement

Adults
- Teeth grinding, chewing issues
- Preventing/treating dental decay and gum care
- Reinforcing teeth brushing/home care
- Restorative dentistry for missing teeth/decayed teeth

CHAPTER 15

Down Syndrome and the Eye—Significance of Early Screening

Leila Mohan

INTRODUCTION

Down syndrome (DS) is the most common chromosomal anomaly seen globally with an extra copy of all or part of chromosome 21. The intellectual and systemic associations have a wide range from near normal to severe involvement. Almost all structures of the eye can be involved to a variable extent, the most common being refractive errors and accommodation deficiencies. Lid abnormalities, nasolacrimal duct obstruction, strabismus, amblyopia, cataract, and keratoconus are frequently seen, and glaucoma, retinal, and optic nerve abnormalities, which are not so common, can affect visual performance significantly. All these ophthalmic conditions are seen more commonly in children with DS than in the general population. Many of the issues, if detected early by screening, can be corrected, giving the child a better quality of life and easier integration into social life. Refractive errors, strabismus, media opacities due to cataract, and keratoconus can lead to amblyopia, which, if not detected and treated early, leads to permanent visual disability.

REFRACTIVE ERRORS

Significant refractive errors are seen in 50–80% of children with DS. There is a failure to emmetropize. A normal child is born hypermetropic. As he grows, the corneal curvature flattens, the axial length of the eyeball increases, the lens flattens, and there is a coordinated growth of all these refractive elements to emmetropize, i.e., to normalize the refractive power. This emmetropization is impaired in DS and is probably the reason for the higher incidence of hypermetropia and oblique astigmatism, which is commonly seen in the normal infant.

In general, children do not complain about their visual disability. The general inattention in children with DS is taken for granted by the parents and physicians. Unless you screen them, the visual disability goes unnoticed. Often, a Teller acuity assessment of visual acuity is possible. In myopia or short sight, the child does not see far objects clearly, and in significant hypermetropia, both near and distant vision may be affected, and the child gives up trying to look for minute details. Large astigmatism where only one axis is affected is also not uncommon. Anisometropia is when there is a large difference in refractive status between the two eyes, when the more ametropic eye (the eye with larger refractive error) can develop amblyopia and strabismus. Both high myopia and high hypermetropia are seen more frequently in children with DS and can be fully corrected with concave or convex lenses, respectively. Astigmatism, i.e., abnormal optical power in one axis of the eye, is not uncommon and is corrected with cylindrical lenses. High myopia not only produces blurring of vision but also leads to retinal degenerative changes, which, if not followed up, can lead to retinal detachment. A simple screening of refractive status, even if the child is not cooperative enough for subjective vision testing, can be done and treated with spectacle correction. Use of spectacles, though not easily accepted, must be encouraged. The visual clarity which it gives is soon made out. Often, parents are reluctant to give glasses to young children, but once they start using them, they find a positive change in visual behavior. So, every child with DS should have a vision screening at least by 1 year of age.

ABNORMALITIES OF ACCOMMODATION

Accommodation is the process by which the eye changes its refractive power when focusing from a far distance to near **(Fig. 1)**.

Though refractive status and accommodation are very closely associated, there is an inherent deficiency in children with DS. About 80% of them are found to underaccommodate for all distances. As refractive errors are common, after correcting the refractive error, a lag of accommodation should be looked for. This is done by the

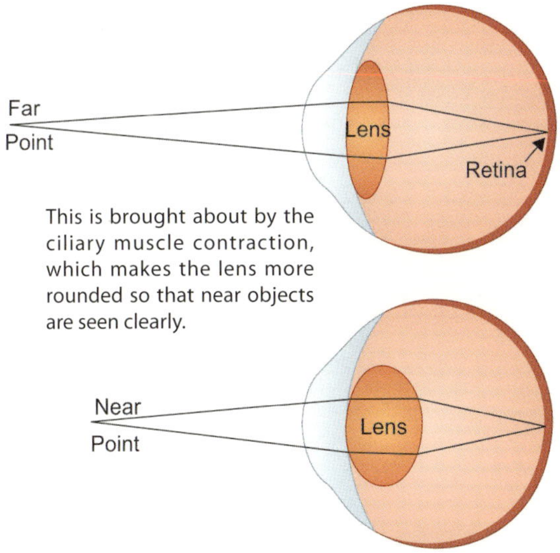

Fig. 1: Accommodation of the eye.

technique of dynamic retinoscopy, i.e., with the glasses in place; retinoscopy is done when the child is focusing for near. As high hypermetropia sets a lot of demand on accommodation to see clearly, there may be an additional blur for focusing for near in these children. A child with uncorrected hypermetropia uses his accommodation to overcome this, which reduces the reserve to focus for near vision. On the other hand, in uncorrected myopia, a child need not have accommodative power for near since he already focuses for near well, though he cannot see clearly for distance. Underaccommodation is common in all types of refractive errors, and a dynamic retinoscopy with the spectacle correction in place is mandatory in these children, especially during school-going age. Lag of accommodation can be treated by giving bifocal spectacles where the child can see far objects through the upper segment and near objects through the lower segment **(Fig. 2)**. They perform better at school when an add lens (bifocal) is given, even when they have no refractive error. Bifocals help children in concentrating on near work at school and also with digital gadgets.

Strabismus

Strabismus or squinting is more prevalent among children with DS. Its prevalence may be as high as 50%. Esotropia or convergent strabismus is the most common type seen by the age of 3–4 years, in contrast to essential infantile esotropia. A pseudoesotropia, due to prominent epicanthus that is commonly seen in these children, gives a false appearance

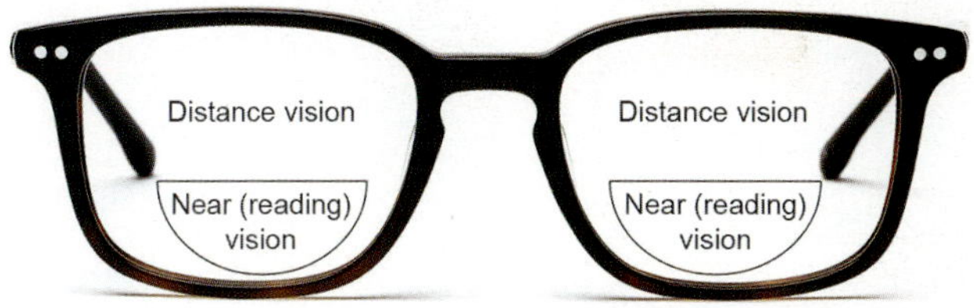

Fig. 2: Bifocal glasses to help accommodate lag for near vision.

of strabismus and should be ruled out. Recent studies show that lag of accommodation and hypermetropia due to impaired emmetropization may be the reason for a higher incidence of esotropia at this age. In an attempt to focus on near, they try to accommodate excessively, which induces more convergence. It is also seen that esotropia in children with DS develops much later, by about 4 years, in contrast to the usual accommodative esotropia which occurs by about 2–3 years. Proper spectacle correction of hypermetropia may prevent or correct the strabismus if treated early. Without treatment, strabismus can lead to strabismic amblyopia, which may impair binocular vision permanently.

Early diagnosis and management by a pediatric ophthalmologist is important. Spectacle correction by itself or patching, if amblyopia has set in, may often correct vision and binocularity. If there is strabismus after correction of refraction, surgical management as in any child is necessary to align the eyes, and attention to refractive correction and amblyopia with patching continued. Hypermetropia reduces over time, and myopia may progress.

Amblyopia

Amblyopia has a higher incidence due to various causes—hypermetropia, oblique astigmatism, anisometropia, strabismus, and optical media opacities such as cataract. Since vision assessment is critical in diagnosing amblyopia, frequent follow-up of refractive status and cataract, if present, is important. Large oblique astigmatism often points to a keratoconus, i.e., progressive ectasia of a conical cornea. When vision in one eye is poor compared to the other eye, a suppression from central neural connections occurs when both eyes are open, the child uses only one eye. Gradually, the vision in the eye which was not used deteriorates further and becomes permanently impaired. A minimal cataract, which is not visually significant, can

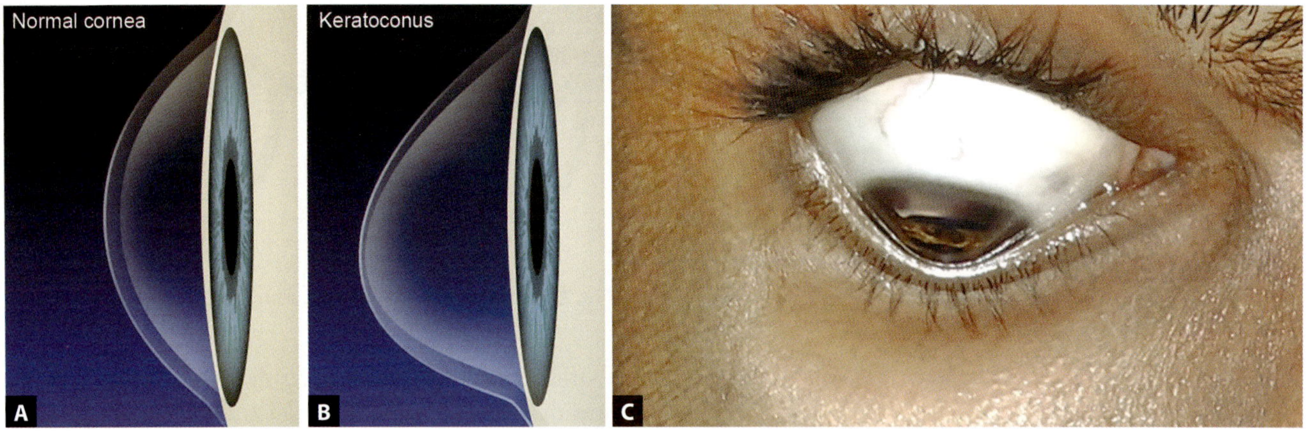

Figs. 3A to C: Keratoconus of the eye.

progress and become visually significant. So, follow-up of cataract is important. Late intervention may lead to amblyopia, i.e., even after cataract surgery, vision may not improve. Underdiagnosis is common since one eye is enough for most activities. Unless frequent follow-up is done and management in the form of spectacles and occlusion (patching—to forcibly use the eye with poor vision) is done, visual impairment becomes permanent. Large ametropia, i.e., high refractive error in both eyes, can also produce ametropic amblyopia in both eyes, if not corrected with glasses.

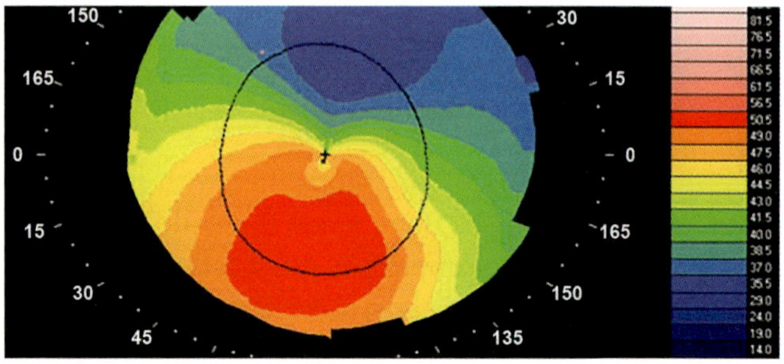

Fig. 4: Corneal topography showing varying curvature of different axes of the cornea.

Keratoconus

Keratoconus is the progressive thinning with conical protrusion of the cornea, impairing vision significantly, especially during adolescent years (**Figs. 3A to C**).

When there is large astigmatism, i.e., increased curvature of only one axis or scissoring of reflexes when doing retinoscopy, keratoconus must be suspected, especially if the axis or power of the cylinder changes over time. This can be detected early by a corneal topography—i.e., mapping of corneal curvature and corneal pachymetry—i.e., measuring the thickness of the central cornea and following them up **(Fig. 4)**.

In advanced cases, corneal hydrops, i.e., sudden breaking of the Descemet's membrane producing waterlogging or acute edema of the cornea and later corneal opacities, can occur. It has been shown that frequent rubbing of the cornea, as in chronic blepharitis, which is common in children with DS, is a causative factor in the progression of keratoconus. The prevalence of keratoconus in various ethnic populations was shown to be 5–36%. In one study, it was as high as 70%, probably due to the criteria taken for diagnosis, as topographic diagnosis detects keratoconus early now. Collagen V1, seen in the cornea, encoded by some genes in chromosome 21, may have a role in producing keratoconus and cardiac problems in DS.

Keratoconus is one of the major indications for corneal transplantation (keratoplast) globally. Early diagnosis provides the opportunity to prevent progression of the ectasia by treatment with collagen cross-linking of the cornea before it advances to the stage requiring corneal transplant. Postoperative management after keratoplasty is very challenging in children with DS. Collagen cross-linking is a procedure by which the cornea is strengthened using UV light and riboflavin, which stiffens the corneal collagen and reduces keratoconus progression. So, screening for refractive error and diagnosing keratoconus early is important.

Nystagmus

Nystagmus is seen in about 30% of children. The majority of them have infantile nystagmus syndrome. A manifest horizontal nystagmus is the most common type, though it can be latent and associated with esotropia. Neuroimaging could not demonstrate any progressive cause for the nystagmus. So it is not mandatory. It has been shown that myopia has a higher prevalence among children with DS having nystagmus than in those who do not have nystagmus. It may need surgical intervention if associated with significant head posture.

Cataract

Blue dot cataracts or cerulean cataracts, which do not affect vision, are quite common among children with DS. Congenital dense cataracts necessitating immediate surgery occur 10 times higher in these children and need early surgical intervention during infancy. Dense cataracts at birth, if not removed by 3 months, lead to dense amblyopia and sensory nystagmus with poor vision. This signifies the importance of early screening, looking for red reflex and referral to the ophthalmologist if necessary. Congenital or acquired cataract has a prevalence of 15% in DS. It has also been shown that cataract in the adult population with DS occur at an earlier age. The visual outcome postoperatively is comparable to that in the general population.

Lid Abnormalities

Eyelid abnormalities are almost universal, with a prevalence of 90%, and are not visually significant. Prominent epicanthal folds (96%), congenital ectropion, entropion, epiblepharon, and ptosis are all reported. Congenital floppy eyelids, with spontaneous eversion of lids during sleep, can rarely be seen and treated conservatively and surgery done, only if necessary.

Blepharoconjunctivitis occurs more frequently in these children and the consequent infections such as chalazion and hordeolum are common. Some attribute this to the slanting palpebral fissure and other lid malpositions and the lower immunity in DS. Another important factor as mentioned is the frequent rubbing due to untreated infection or inflammation, which can predispose to the causation or progression of keratoconus.

Congenital Nasolacrimal Duct Obstruction

Nasolacrimal duct obstruction (NLDO) with chronic dacryocystitis is a common occurrence in children with DS with a prevalence of 22%. Though conventionally, it is due to obstruction at the valve of Hasner **(Fig. 5)**, the facial morphologic features may contribute to the higher incidence of NLDO, and canalicular abnormalities may be associated. It presents with watering, discharge, and stickiness of eyelids since birth, and often there is matting of eyelashes at presentation. It may be bilateral or unilateral. Conservative management with a mild antibiotic eye drop for the infection and hydrostatic massaging over the lacrimal sac area (Crigler maneuver) **(Fig. 6)**, if done efficiently clear the obstruction in 85% of the cases. Attention should be given to any nasal pathology too and crusting inside the nose is prevented by the use of saline nasal drops. After 8–10 months, the chance of spontaneous resolution is less and probing to open up the obstruction has to be considered by 1 year of age. In children awaiting cataract surgery, this may need to be done earlier. When primary probing fails, silicon intubation may be necessary.

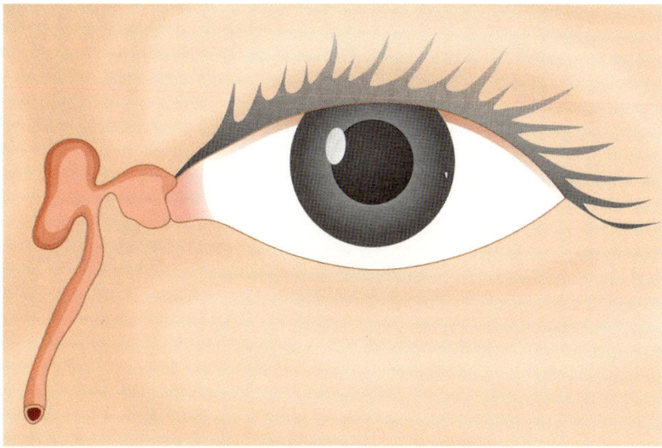

Fig. 5: Nasolacrimal duct obstruction.

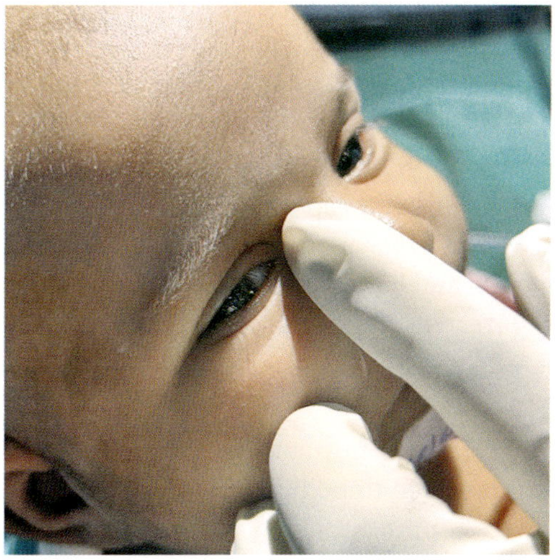

Fig. 6: Crigler massage.

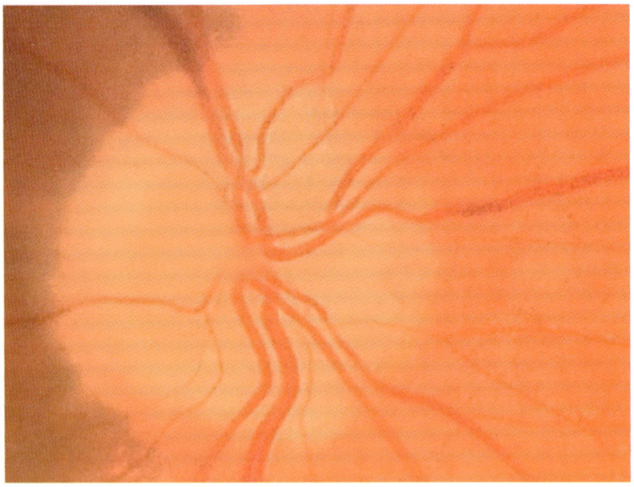

Fig. 7: Optic nerve head drusen.

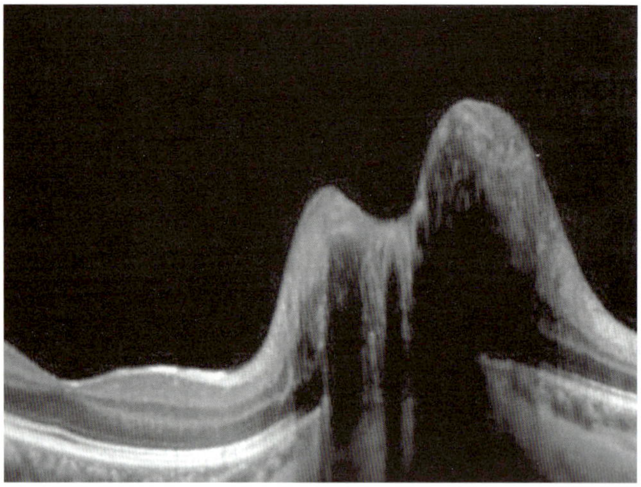

Fig. 8: Optical coherence tomography (OCT) imaging of ONHD.

When watering or epiphora occurs with photophobia and pain, glaucoma has to be suspected and evaluated.

Recently a higher incidence of anisometropic amblyopia has been reported in children with NLDO, and they need to have a comprehensive examination at presentation and be followed up till 2–3 years to consider optical correction with spectacles if necessary.

Glaucoma

Glaucoma, though not common in children with DS, has been reported to be higher. A child presenting with watery eyes, photophobia, and blepharospasm has to be investigated to rule out glaucoma; if necessary, an examination under anesthesia for IOP and corneal Haab's striae. Angle surgery has been shown to be more challenging in these cases than in primary congenital glaucoma.

RETINAL AND OPTIC NERVE PATHOLOGY

Retinal abnormalities are seen in about 2–40% of children. Optic disc abnormalities are common. Abnormal vasculature over the disc giving a crowded appearance is very common. Peripapillary atrophy giving a myopic appearance is also very common. Tortuosity of vessels, increased thickness of retinal nerve fiber layer, and optic nerve head drusen (ONHD) are some of the abnormalities seen more in DS, which do not affect vision adversely. ONHD **(Fig. 7)** may mimic a disc edema and can be easily differentiated now by optical coherence tomography (OCT) imaging **(Fig. 8)**.

Retinal detachment can occur more frequently and may be traumatic in nature due to self-inflicted injuries and may present late. Due to the late presentation, the surgical outcome may be poor.

OTHER OCULAR FEATURES

Brushfield spots—they are small, benign, white, gray, or yellow spots that appear in a circular pattern around the iris's edge. It is due to hyperplasia of iris stromal connective tissue, which is more commonly appreciated in blue irides.

Anesthesia Considerations

Planning of anesthesia and perioperative management should be customised in children with DS.

CONCLUSION

Children with DS have a higher incidence of ocular involvement, which may impair vision. Most of these conditions if detected early can be treated successfully. Since 80% of learning and social interaction in children are from visual feedback, awareness of these abnormalities and timely referral and rehabilitation is important.

SUGGESTED READING

1. Adio AO, Wajuihian SO. Ophthalmic manifestations of children with Down syndrome in Port Harcourt, Nigeria. Clin Ophthalmol. 2012;6:1859-64.
2. Akoto T, Li JJ, Estes AJ, Karamichos D, Liu Y. The Underlying Relationship between Keratoconus and Down Syndrome. Intl J Mol Sci. 2022;23(18):10796.

3. AlAhmadi BO, Alsulaiman SM, Arevalo JF. Retinal Detachment in Down Syndrome: Characteristics and Surgical Outcome. Ophthalmol. 2016;2016:6971591.
4. Areaux RG, Sorenson S, Childhood glaucoma in Down syndrome, Journal of American Association for Pediatric Ophthalmology and Strabismus, 2021,25(4):e14, https://doi.org/10.1016/j.jaapos.2021.08.055.
5. Averbuch-Heller L, Dell'Osso LF, Jacobs JB, Remler BF. Latent and congenital nystagmus in Down syndrome. J Neuroophthalmol. 1999:19:166-72.
6. Berk AT, Saatci AO, Erçal MD, Tunç M, Ergin M. Ocular findings in 55 patients with Down's syndrome. Ophthalmic Genet. 1996:17(1):15-9.
7. Cregg M, Woodhouse JM, Pakeman VH, Saunders KJ, Gunter HL, Parker M, et al. Accommodation and refractive error in children with Down syndrome: cross-sectional and longitudinal studies. Invest Ophthalmol Vis Sci. 2001 Jan;42(1):55-63. PMID: 11133848.
8. de Weger C, Boonstra N, Goossens J. Bifocals reduce strabismus in children with Down syndrome: Evidence from a randomized controlled trial. Acta Ophthalmol. 2020; 98:89-97.
9. Dumitrescu AV, Moga DC, Longmuir SQ, Olson RJ, Drack AV. Prevalence and Characteristics of Abnormal Head Posture in children with Down syndrome - a 20 year retrospective, descriptive review. Ophthalmology. 2011; 118(9):1859-64.
10. Haseeb A, Huynh E, ElSheikh RH, ElHawary AS, Scelfo C, Ledoux DM, et al. Down syndrome: a review of ocular manifestations. Ther Adv Ophthalmol. 2022;14: 25158414221101718.
11. Jaeger EA. Ocular findings in Down's syndrome. Trans Am Ophth Soc. 1980:78:808-45.
12. Kazemi M, Salehi M, Kheirollahi M. Down Syndrome: Current Status, Challenges and Future Perspectives. Int J Mol Cell Med. 2016 Summer;5(3):125-33.
13. Krinsky-McHale SJ, Jenkins EC, Zigman WB, Silverman W. Ophthalmic disorders in adults with Down Syndrome. Curr Gerontol Geriatric Res. 2012;2012:974253.
14. Kristianslund O, Drolsum L. Prevalence of keratoconus in persons with Down syndrome: a review. BMJ Open Ophthalmol. 2021;6(1):e000754.
15. Lin AE, Chang YC, Lin MY, Tam KW, Shen YD. Comparison of treatment for congenital nasolacrimal duct obstruction: a systematic review and meta-analysis. Can J Ophthalmol. 2016;51(1):34-40.
16. Marilyn J. Bull, the Committee on Genetics; Health Supervision for Children With Down Syndrome. Pediatrics August 2011;128(2):393-406. 10.1542/peds.2011-1605
17. Matta NS, Singman EL, Silbert DI. Prevalence of amblyopia risk factors in congenital nasolacrimal duct obstruction. J AAPOS. 2010;14(5):386-8.
18. Najmi H, Mobarki Y, Mania K, Altowairqi B, Basehi M, Mahfouz MS, et al. The correlation between keratoconus and eye rubbing: A Review. Int J Ophthalmol. 2019;12:1775-81.
19. Ugurlu A, Altinkurt E. Ophthalmologic Manifestations and Retinal Findings in Children with Down Syndrome. J Ophthalmol. 2020;2020:9726261.
20. Umfress AC, Hair CD, Donahue SP. Prevalence of Ocular Pathology on Initial Screening and Incidence of New Findings on Follow-up Examinations in Children with Trisomy 21. Am J Ophthalmol. 2019;207:373-7.
21. Wong MM, Schneier AJ, Ledoux D, Heidary G. Neuroimaging findings in patients with down syndrome and nystagmus. J Pediatr Ophthalmol Strabismus. 2016:53:383.
22. Woodhouse JM, Cregg M, Gunter HL, Sanders DP, Saunders KJ, Pakeman VH, et al. The effect of age, size of target and cognitive factors on accommodative responses of children with Down syndrome. Invest Ophthalmol Vis Sci. 2000;41:2479-85.
23. Zahidi AAA, McIlreavy L, Erichsen JT, Woodhouse JM. Visual and Refractive Status of Children with Down's Syndrome and Nystagmus. IOVS. 2022;63(2):28.

CHAPTER 16

Down Syndrome: Otolaryngological Manifestations

Manoj MP

INTRODUCTION

Down syndrome (DS) presents a serious challenge to the otolaryngologist, as >50% of them are likely to be affected with ear, nose, and throat complaints during their lifetime. There is clear evidence that ENT interventions such as laryngoscopy, audiometry, tracheostomy, tympanoplasty, or mastoidectomy are performed much more in individuals with DS than those without.

COMMON CONDITIONS REQUIRING ENT INTERVENTIONS

As it is seen in **Table 1**, an otolaryngologist should be recruited early into the initial evaluation and management of this condition. A recommended screening schedule is to be followed **(Table 2)** and primary care physicians are required to follow this with all care and concern that essential interventions are not delayed.

TABLE 1: Conditions requiring ENT intervention.

Otologic concern	*Oral/nasal/pharyngeal*	*Airway*	*Systemic*
Narrow ear canals	Obstructive sleep apnea	Laryngomalacia	Hypotonia
Low-set ears	Low and wide nasal bridge	Subglottic stenosis	Obesity
Eustachian tube block	Short palate	Complete tracheal rings	Thyroid disorders
Chronic otitis media	Facial hypoplasia	Tracheal bronchus	Immunodeficiency
Hearing loss	Rhinorrhea, congestion	Vascular compression	Neurodevelopmental delay
Cochlear anomalies	Hypoplastic sinuses	Tracheomalacia	Cervical spine instability
Vestibular anomalies	Enlarged tonsils and adenoids	Laryngeal cleft	ADHD
Cochlear nerve deficiency	Large and protruded tongue	Dysphagia and aspiration	Anemia

(ADHD: attention deficit hyperactivity disorder)

TABLE 2: Timing of screening.

Screening	*First 30 days*	*1–12 months*	*1–5 years*	*6–13 years*	*13–21 years*
Hearing	Screening +ABR	Confirm screening + ABR	Audiogram every 6 months until normal and then yearly if symptomatic	Annual audiogram if symptomatic	Annual audiogram if symptomatic
Swallow	Screening if symptomatic, video fluoroscopy and feeding evaluation	NR	NR	NR	NR
Sleep quality	NR	Screening for OSA, PSG if indicated	Annual screening for OSA, PSG at 3–4 years	Annual screening	Annual screening
Airway function	Screen for noisy breathing	NR	NR	NR	NR

(ABR: auditory brainstem response; OSA: obstructive sleep apnea; PSG: polysomnography)

There is, over a period, a substantial increase in the lifespan of individuals with DS and there is a high probability that more office visits to the otolaryngologists will happen in the later years. Hence, these screening protocols need to be strictly enforced so that overall quality of life improvement is possible.

OTOLOGIC CONSIDERATIONS

External Auditory Canal Issues

The position of the pinna and very narrow external auditory canals (EAC) are some of the most defining characteristics of DS. EAC stenosis is found in >50% of people with this condition. It is important that periodic cleaning of the canal is done to prevent the accumulation of wax and debris, leading to significant conductive hearing loss. Children need cleaning of the canal under the microscope every 3–6 months as an office procedure. It also needs an efficient clinician to perform this as these children are very sensitive to pain and any discomfort will reduce cooperation. Wax and debris removal is not only useful to improve hearing but also to facilitate hearing monitoring and prevent the development of middle ear infections.

Eustachian Tube Block

It is said that children with DS are much more likely to develop eustachian tube blockage than other children of the same age because their tubes are often collapsed, narrow, and straight **(Fig. 1)**. Adding to the problem are other associations of DS—midface hypoplasia, adenoid enlargement, and increased upper respiratory infections. The high incidence of middle ear effusion (MEE) and otitis media with effusion (OME) among individuals with DS is well established; it has been reported that the prevalence of OME at 12 months of age was 93% and at 5 years, it was 68%. Conductive hearing loss is present in up to 80% of children with DS with OME, making treatment of MEE paramount to prevent adverse effects on language development. We find that sensorineural hearing loss (SNHL) too is found at a rate slightly higher than an age-matched control of children without DS. Though the American Academy of Pediatrics (AAP) recommends that all children be screened for hearing loss before 3 months of age, hearing assessment in children with DS is recommended every 6 months until the age of 3–4 even if they pass the newborn screening. A 2012 study by Park and colleagues found that 26.2% of 332 patients with DS did not pass a newborn hearing test. Although most of the hearing loss was conductive owing to serous MEE, a smaller percentage of the patients had both SNHL (1.5%) and mixed hearing loss (MHL) (1%). There is another subset of children with hearing loss due to cochlear dysplasia and/or deficient cochlear nerves.

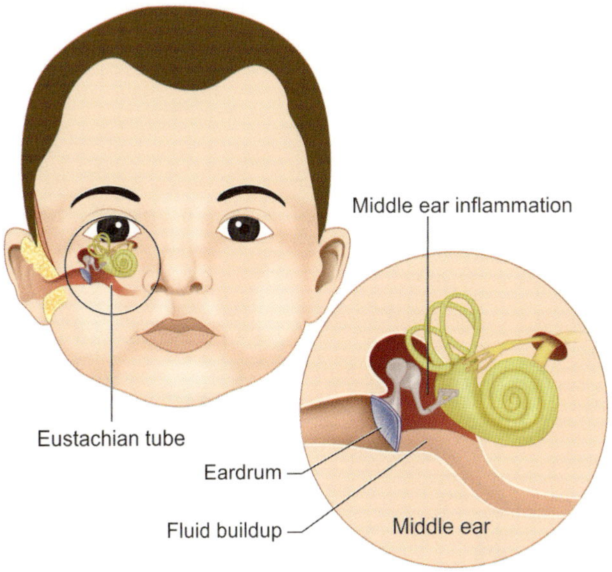

Fig. 1: Eustachian tube block in Down syndrome causing otitis media.

Intervention strategies for children with hearing disorders depend upon the cause. Conductive hearing loss due to MEE is the most common cause and may need ventilation tube insertion according to the guidelines for this procedure in other children. There could be technical difficulties in ventilation tube placement due to the narrow eustachian tube and in such cases, careful surveillance and later placement of tubes may be considered if there is no further detriment to hearing **(Fig. 2)**. The timing of ventilation tube placement is the usual 3 months after a trial of medical management and it is preferred to use titanium ventilation tubes for longer persistence and decreased chance of postventilation tube otorrhea.

Even after the ventilation tube is placed, monitoring of hearing progress must be made over the ensuing years, and sometimes repetition of the procedure may be needed. Failure to place ventilation tubes may result in adhesion of the tympanic membrane to the middle ear, called adhesive otitis media, and result in permanent hearing loss and cholesteatoma. As in normal children, recurrence of middle ear fluid may necessitate adenoid surgery or endoscopic sinus surgery on the failure of myringotomy procedure. Our protocol has been to monitor middle ear function and the presence of fluid.

Then, if the child is allergic, inhaled nasal corticosteroids (INCS) are started and tympanometry is repeated after 3 months. If effusion is still present, a ventilation tube is inserted under general anesthesia. After this, the audiogram is repeated every month and the middle ear function, which cannot be monitored with the ventilation tube, is tested after the grommet extrudes in about a year. A proportion of children develop recurrence of MEE and if so, a longer-lasting tube like the T tube is inserted and if there is significant mouth breathing, and inability to taper INCS, then adenoidectomy is considered, albeit with lesser evidence.

For children with more severe hearing loss, hearing aids are an option but there are inherent difficulties in fitting aids in very narrow canals. If the hearing loss is purely conductive, or if there is a mixed component, bone conduction hearing devices or implants are legitimate options. Devices such as Contact Mini, BAHA (bone-anchored hearing aid) soft band, and Adhear offer nonsurgical solutions for this category of people **(Figs. 3A to C)**.

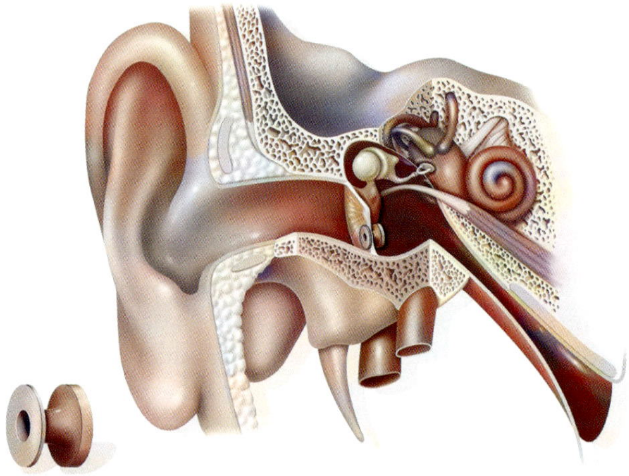

Fig. 2: Ventilation tube placement in middle ear effusion to prevent complications.

An implantable solution is also at hand, where these bone conduction devices are fixed onto the bone behind the ear with screws and provide superior hearing characteristics. Among these are BAHA, Bone Bridge. and OSIA (osseointegrated steady-state implant) **(Figs. 4A to C)**. They are expensive options but provide superior performance with better cosmetic appeal. Unfortunately, government funding for implants is not available in many countries for children with conductive losses unlike those with sensorineural loss. Organizations who aid and support DS should represent to their respective government to ensure that early and timely funding is given to those in need.

Profound SNHL is not unheard of in DS. In the last 10 years, eight children have presented with severe to profound hearing loss to the author and two of them have opted for cochlear implant surgery. A prerequisite is a child who is intellectually able to cooperate with therapy sessions, parents who are willing to accept the outcomes and a surgical and habilitation team who are skilled enough to take on this challenging job. Surgery is no different from other children without comorbidities, but there may be anesthesia concerns that cause a slightly increased risk, but not so much that it is contraindicated.

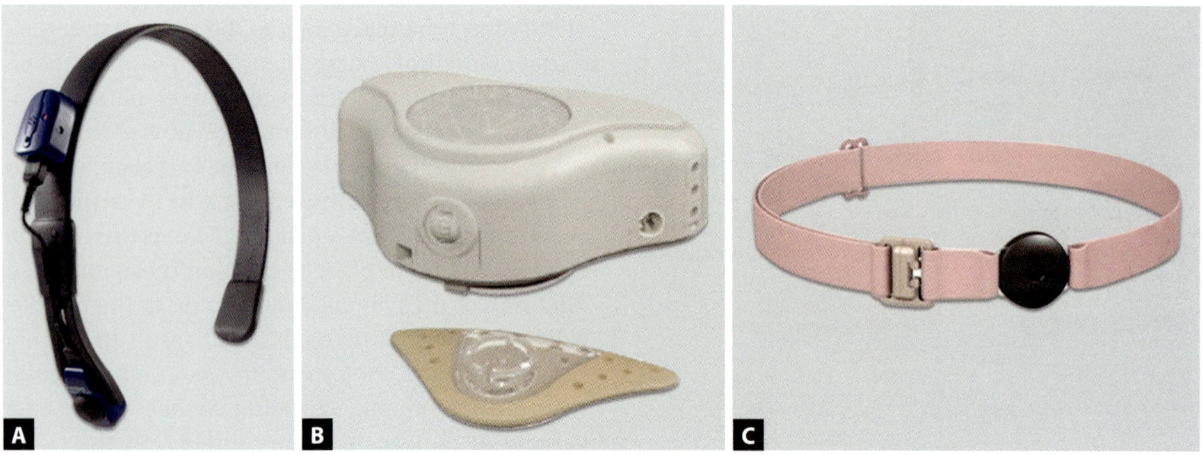

Contact mini — Adhear — BAHA soft band

Figs. 3A to C: Nonimplantable bone conduction hearing devices.

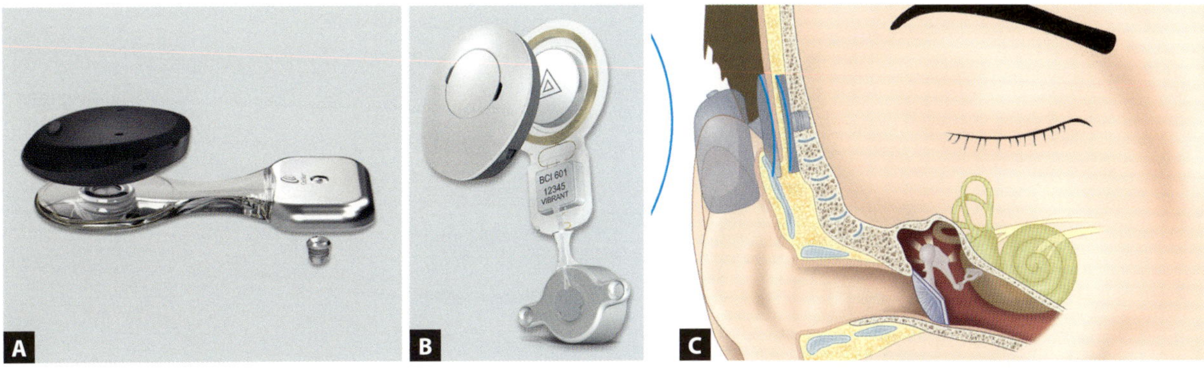

Cochlear osia Bone bridge medel Cochlear BAHA

Figs. 4A to C: Implantable bone conduction hearing devices.

SINUSITIS AND UPPER AIRWAY INFECTIONS

DS is characterized by midface hypoplasia, narrow nasal passages, and hypoplastic sinuses. These predispose to nasal obstruction, discharge and chronic rhinosinusitis, adenoid hypertrophy, ciliary dysfunction, and immune compromise. These mostly require only primary care, sometimes nasal irrigation, INCS, and occasional antibiotics for infections, but occasionally need adeno-idectomy or endoscopic sinus surgery. It must be noted that the recurrence of adenoids is much more in DS than in an age-matched normal control of the population.

SLEEP, AIRWAY, AND SWALLOWING

Obstructive sleep apnea (OSA) is a frequently seen symptom of DS. This accounts for most of the visits to otolaryngologists and it is estimated that up to 80% of children with DS compared to 2–4% in a typical population. AAP recommends screening by polysomnography (PSG) in children with DS at 3–4 years of age. Memory loss, cognitive impairment, and systemic medical comorbidities are seen in many patients with OSA and DS is no different. However, the risk of pulmonary hypertension is high in untreated OSA and as they age, narrowing of the airway further compounds this problem.

Pediatric patients with DS have many anatomical risk factors for OSA. Adenotonsillar hypertrophy is common in these patients, as are craniofacial abnormalities including midface and mandibular hypoplasia, narrow nasopharynx, macroglossia, shortened palate, and lingual tonsil hypertrophy that may predispose them to upper airway obstruction. Patients with DS may also have generalized hypotonia that contributes to glossoptosis, hypopharyngeal collapse, and laryngomalacia. Furthermore, children with DS who are also obese are twice as likely as other children with DS to have OSA, which at baseline is more severe.

Treatment of OSA in children with DS includes adenotonsillectomy, positive airway pressure (PAP), tracheostomy and hypoglossal nerve stimulators. Adenotonsillectomy, though very effective in reducing OSA, must be attempted with caution, as complications of this surgery, viz., bleeding, increased hospitalizations, anesthesia complications, and recurrence of OSA are much more common than in children without DS.

Positive airway pressure is useful in those not willing for surgery, very obese, or surgical failures. Compliance is difficult to achieve and the use of nasal prongs may be useful than traditional masks. It is said that compliance rates vary from 56% to 81% in various studies, only slightly less than in a normal population. The hypoglossal nerve stimulator is an exciting discovery and is now medically approved for use. The high cost of surgery and maintenance is a huge limiting factor in many countries but costs are expected to reduce over time. The hypoglossal nerve stimulator (Inspire Medical Systems) is a surgically implantable device that uses a sensor electrode in the intercostal muscles and a stimulation lead around anterior branches of the hypoglossal nerve to deliver electrical impulses to tongue protrusion muscles during inspiration to alleviate tongue base obstruction during sleep **(Figs. 5A and B)**.

Criteria for implantation of the hypoglossal nerve stimulator in children with DS are currently strict:

- 10–20 years of age
- Medically stable with a body mass index <32

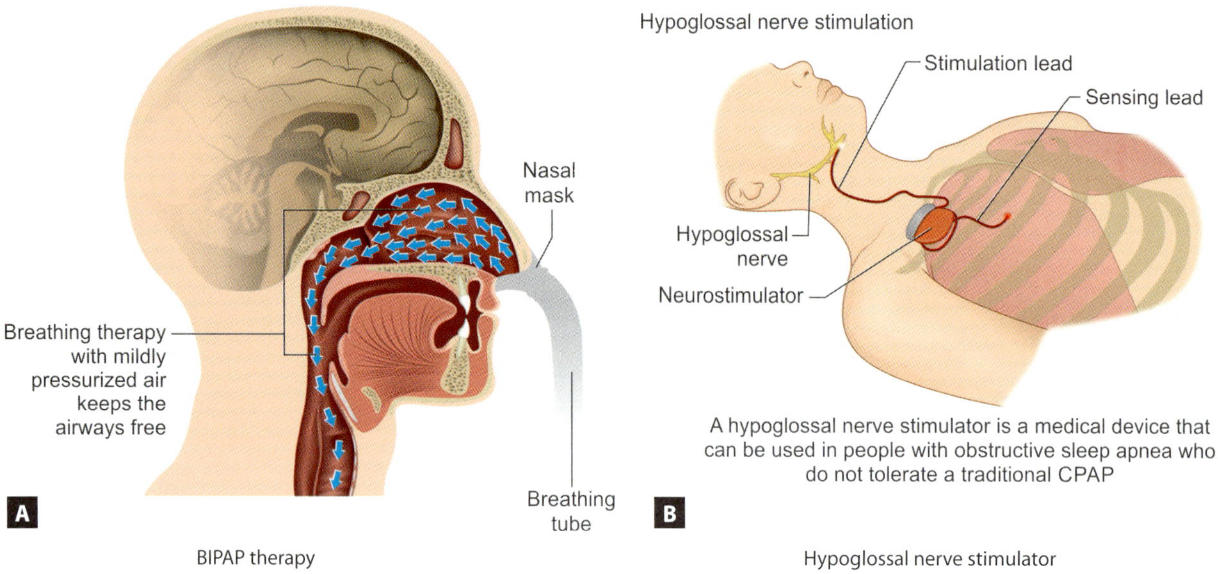

Figs. 5A and B: Intervention for Obstructive sleep apnea. (BIPAP: bilevel positive airway pressure)

- PSG within 6 months demonstrating severe persistent OSA with apnea-hypopnea index between 10 and 50 events/h.

In addition, drug-induced sleep endoscopy (DISE) must not show circumferential collapse at the level of the velopharynx.

In adults who have DS and OSA, BIPAP appliances are the cornerstone of therapy, though compliance issues as in children are common. One of the most important reasons why adult OSA is to be identified and treated is that they hardly complain, despite having severe daytime sleepiness and fatigue. They have an increased risk anyway of premature aging, depression, and dementia and this can be worsened with severe OSA. A hypoglossal nerve stimulator is an option, as in children, with the mentioned drawbacks of cost and availability.

Airway Problems in Down Syndrome

Laryngomalacia, laryngotracheal cleft, tracheomalacia, subglottic stenosis (congenital and acquired), tracheal stenosis, complete tracheal rings, and tracheal bronchus complicate the airway issues in DS. Presenting symptoms may include stridor, dyspnea, cough, recurrent respiratory infections, aspiration, and/or cyanosis or apnea. Laryngomalacia may persist beyond infancy because of hypotonia and gastroesophageal reflux. Supraglottoplasty, an effective procedure for laryngomalacia is fraught with danger in these patients, with failure to relieve symptoms, respiratory distress, need for tracheostomy, and increased mortality.

Congenital subglottic stenosis is common in DS and is 10 times higher than in general population. Therefore, if intubation is needed in DS, it is imperative that a smaller size endotracheal tube to be inserted for it can lead to necrosis and stenosis. Symptomatic and asymptomatic tracheal and subglottic stenosis is also seen and may need surgical intervention.

SWALLOWING DIFFICULTIES

Individuals with DS may experience challenges with swallowing and feeding, which can be related to oral motor skills and coordination. Children are at increased risk of swallowing disorders and aspiration which may continue into adulthood. Anatomic factors, such as shortened palate, macroglossia, dental anomalies, and airway anomalies as previously described along with functional deficits, including hypotonia and delayed development of oromotor function increase the risk of an unsafe swallow in this population. Underlying immune deficiency in the setting of aspiration events may predispose patients with DS to a greater risk of pneumonia and recurrent infections.

The issues that most people with DS face such as picky eating, stuffing food, and excessively slow or rapid rate of eating will all predispose them to aspiration pneumonia and choking. Working with a speech therapist or feeding specialist can help address these issues and early referrals are necessary for preventing complications.

Therefore, it is important to realize the role of the otolaryngologist in managing children and adults with DS. It starts on the day of birth and continues throughout life. As life expectancy and mainstreaming of these people continue to improve, proper and appropriate care and monitoring by the ENT surgeon greatly improve quality of life and reduce morbidity. The primary caregivers and pediatricians should also appreciate this fact and make way for early referral and collaboration with the otolaryngologist so that this goal is achieved.

SPEECH DISORDERS

Individuals with DS may experience various speech and language difficulties, including articulation problems, expressive language delays, and receptive language difficulties. Common speech disorders in individuals with DS include:

- *Articulation disorders:* Some individuals with DS may have difficulty producing certain speech sounds accurately due to differences in oral structures and muscle tone. This can result in unclear speech and difficulty in being understood by others.
- *Expressive language delays:* Individuals with DS may have delays in developing expressive language skills, such as using words to communicate wants and needs, sharing thoughts and ideas, and forming complete sentences. This can lead to challenges in expressing themselves effectively.
- *Receptive language difficulties:* Some individuals may face challenges in understanding and processing language, including following directions, comprehending complex sentences, and grasping abstract concepts. This can impact their ability to comprehend and interact effectively in various social and academic settings.
- *Apraxia of speech:* Few individuals with DS may also experience apraxia of speech, a neurological disorder that affects the ability to plan and coordinate the movements needed for speech. This can result in inconsistent speech errors, difficulty producing speech sounds in sequence, and overall reduced intelligibility.

Treatment for speech disorders in individuals with DS typically involves speech therapy provided by a qualified speech-language pathologist. Therapy focuses on improving speech sound production, enhancing language skills, increasing vocabulary and comprehension, and promoting overall communication abilities. Family involvement and ongoing practice are also crucial in supporting and enhancing communication skills in individuals with DS.

CONCLUSION

With over half of the children with DS presenting with Otolaryngological manifestations, closer coordination between the Pediatrician and Otolaryngologist is needed for better outcomes. Early intervention for hearing disorders is crucial in preventing lifelong disability. Conductive, mixed and sensorineural hearing loss is not uncommon, and it requires diligent monitoring to prevent progression. With multiple methods available to correct nearly all these conditions, caregivers must be aware of this and seek treatment at the earliest opportunity. Peculiar anthropomorphic characteristics predispose individuals to sinus infections, as well as breathing and swallowing difficulties. Snoring is common in children with DS and can lead to multiple problems, including depression and dementia as they get older. Recent technological advances are practical, albeit expensive, and can correct these issues; no effort should be spared, as significant quality of life improvements can result. Swallowing and speech disorders, though not life-threatening, need active intervention by therapists to improve overall well-being. Therefore, the importance of Otorhinolaryngologists' involvement is stressed and needs to go many notches above what is present to make a difference in the lives of these individuals.

SUGGESTED READING

1. Chamseddin BH, Johnson RF, Mitchell RB. Obstructive Sleep Apnea in Children with Down Syndrome: Demographic, Clinical, and Polysomnographic Features. Otolaryngol Head Neck Surg. 2019;160(1):150-7.
2. De Schrijver L, Topsakal V, Wojciechowski M, Van de Heyning P, Boudewyns A. Prevalence and etiology of sensorineural hearing loss in children with down syndrome: A cross-sectional study. Int J Pediatr Otorhinolaryngol. 2019; 116:168-72.
3. Diercks GR, Wentland C, Keamy D, Kinane TB, Skotko B, de Guzman V, et al. Hypoglossal Nerve Stimulation in Adolescents With Down Syndrome and Obstructive Sleep Apnea. JAMA Otolaryngol Head Neck Surg. 2018;144(1): 37-42.

4. Dyken ME, Lin-Dyken DC, Poulton S, Zimmerman MB, Sedars E. Prospective polysomnographic analysis of obstructive sleep apnea in down syndrome. Arch Pediatr Adolesc Med. 2003;157(7):655-60.
5. Farhood Z, Isley JW, Ong AA, Nguyen SA, Camilon TJ, LaRosa AC, et al. Adenotonsillectomy outcomes in patients with Down syndrome and obstructive sleep apnea. Laryngoscope. 2017;127(6):1465-70.
6. Hamilton J, Yaneza MM, Clement WA, Kubba H. The prevalence of airway problems in children with Down's syndrome. Int J Pediatr Otorhinolaryngol. 2016;81:1-4.
7. Jackson A, Maybee J, Moran MK, Wolter-Warmerdam K, Hickey F. Clinical Characteristics of Dysphagia in Children with Down Syndrome. Dysphagia. 2016;31(5):663-71.
8. Kent RD, Vorperian HK. Speech impairment in Down syndrome: A review. J Speech Lang Hear Res. 2013;56(1): 178-210.
9. Lazenby T. The impact of aging on eating, drinking, and swallowing function in people with Down's syndrome. Dysphagia. 2008;23(1):88-97.
10. McDermott AL, Williams J, Kuo MJ, Reid AP, Proops DW. The role of bone anchored hearing aids in children with Down syndrome. Int J Pediatr Otorhinolaryngol. 2008 Jun;72(6):751-7.
11. Miller R, Gray SD, Cotton RT, Myer CM 3rd, Netterville J. Subglottic stenosis and Down syndrome. Am J Otolaryngol. 1990;11(4):274-7.
12. Park AH, Wilson MA, Stevens PT, Harward R, Hohler N. Identification of hearing loss in pediatric patients with Down syndrome. Otolaryngol Head Neck Surg. 2012;146(1): 135-40.
13. Patel TA, Nguyen SA, White DR. Down Syndrome as an indicator for pediatric otolaryngologic procedures. Int J Pediatr Otorhinolaryngol. 2018;112:182-7.
14. Piatti G, Allegra L, Ambrosetti U, De Santi MM. Nasal ciliary function and ultrastructure in Down syndrome. Laryngoscope. 2001;111(7):1227-30.
15. Rosenfeld RM, Tunkel DE, Schwartz SR, Anne S, Bishop CE, Chelius DC, et al. Clinical Practice Guideline: Tympanostomy Tubes in Children (Update). Otolaryngol Head Neck Surg. 2022;166(1_suppl):S1-S55.
16. Shott SR, Joseph A, Heithaus D. Hearing loss in children with Down syndrome. Int J Pediatr Otorhinolaryngol. 2001; 61(3):199-205.
17. Tsou AY, Bulova P, Capone G, Chicoine B, Gelaro B, Harville TO, et al. Medical Care of Adults With Down Syndrome: A Clinical Guideline. JAMA. 2020;324(15):1543-56.
18. Verhulst S. Long Term Continuous Positive Airway Pressure and Non-invasive Ventilation in Obstructive Sleep Apnea in Children With Obesity and Down Syndrome. Front Pediatr. 2020;8:534.
19. Zalzal HG, Lawlor CM. Down Syndrome for the Otolaryngologist: A Review. JAMA Otolaryngol Head Neck Surg. 2023;149(4):360-7.

CHAPTER 17

Puberty, Sexuality, and Management of Menstrual Cycles

Gayathri K

INTRODUCTION

Gonadal insufficiency is a well-known feature of Down syndrome (DS). Boys with DS have an increased risk of both congenital and acquired cryptorchidism. Hypergonadotropic hypogonadism and impaired migration of the spermatic cord along the path of the gubernaculum and impaired cord elongation are the reasons for this. Males with an extra chromosome or autosome are expected to present primary hypogonadism at puberty owing to meiotic germ cell failure. In trisomy 21, primary hypogonadism involves a combined dysfunction of Sertoli and Leydig cells. Hypergonadotropic hypogonadism is present in infancy and progresses throughout late puberty to adulthood in men.

Despite the gonadal dysfunction, puberty is expected to occur on time, and progress at a typical rate as other children. This emphasizes the need to counsel the caregivers to prepare children for upcoming pubertal changes. Though hypogonadism is present, the belief that these people are infertile is untrue as both men and women with DS have fathered and mothered children. Hence, it is important to have an open discussion with adolescents and adults with DS about sexuality and parenthood.

The physical and emotional effects of puberty occur in the same way as in other children. The stages of puberty are same as in other children. In girls, breast development starts first (age range 8–13 years) followed by pubic hair growth, then the first period. The average age for first period in girls with DS is 12 years 6 months (general population it is 13 years). Periods often begin 2 years after the start of breast development. For boys, it is initially the growth of testicles (9–14 years), then growth of penis, followed by pubic hair growth from 10 years of age. Thyroid problems which occur more commonly in these individuals may also affect the timing of puberty.

SEXUALITY

It is important that vulnerable children, young people, and adults are protected; but this should not be at the cost of respecting their human need to love and to be loved, to have friends and to express their sexuality (in ways that suit them and which are acceptable). People with intellectual disability have the right to express their emotions and sexuality and to develop relationships.

All individuals regardless of disability are sexual beings. In the past, sexuality was not considered an issue for young people with DS because of the inaccurate belief that mental retardation was equivalent to permanent childhood. In fact, all people with DS, do have intimacy needs and sexual feelings. The emergence of sexual behavior in the individual with DS alarms, some parents and caretakers who may rightly fear that their child's cognitive defect makes them vulnerable to unwanted pregnancy, sexual exploitation, abuse, and to sexually transmitted diseases.

Individuals with DS need individualized instruction and education to develop appropriate sociosexual behavior. Individuals with DS require routine reproductive health services recommended for the general population including urological care for men, gynecological care for women, and preventive medical services. Education and counseling to prevent unplanned pregnancy, abuse, and sexually transmitted disease should be part of the routine medical care and education for individuals with DS. All individuals with DS have the right to develop and express sexuality in an emotionally satisfying and socially appropriate manner. Teaching children which parts of their body are private and how to stay safe is essential, as is ensuring they know whom they can talk to at home or school if they feel sad or worried.

FERTILITY

Significantly impaired fertility of both sexes is evident in the DS population. Men with DS have lower fertility, but 70% of women with DS are fertile. However, there is an increased chance of miscarriage. There is a 50% chance of having a child with DS with a high chance of having a child other congenital anomalies. Mosaic DS can be associated with fertility in males as the germ cell line can contain normal cells. The dysfunction of Sertoli and Leydig cells is evidenced by the increased production of luteinizing hormone (LH) and follicle-stimulating hormone (FSH), along with the decreased production of anti-Müllerian hormone (AMH). Other studies have shown that the sperm count in men with DS is abnormally low and the resulting azoospermia or oligospermia may be associated with damaged spermatogenesis. In men with DS after puberty the testicular volume falls, the production of gonadotropin rises and gonadal dysfunction worsens with age. Premature menopause in women with DS will reduce their ability to conceive a child at the desired time. Premature ovarian failure might be associated with a reduced ovarian reserve due to oogenesis failure and/or lower levels of primordial cell maturation.

MANAGEMENT OF MENSTRUAL CYCLES

They should be educated about periods in advance so that they know whom to go and what to do. Most girls will be able to cope independently with their periods, but they initially may need some support. They should be educated about sanitary hygiene and should be trained to use sanitary pads. Periods can take between 1 and 2 years to settle down into a regular pattern. Once they settle down, then it occurs in the usual regular pattern. Simple measures to treat dysmenorrhea should be taught to the caregivers. They may also experience premenstrual symptoms, but it may be difficult for women with learning disability to report these symptoms. These symptoms can be variable in severity. Even if they are very mild they can affect a woman's ability to function in many ways. Keeping a diary of behavior and mood can be helpful to identify timing of symptoms in relation to periods. Hence parents/caregivers should be aware of these mood changes and measures taken if needed. Hormonal treatments can be used to treat these premenstrual symptoms. Except in very few cases, it is not advisable to use medical treatment to stop periods before they have started.

Available Treatments

- *Mefenamic acid:* It is an anti-inflammatory medication which can help reduce pain during periods. It should not be used in women with heart failure, asthma, or kidney problems and should not be used under the age of 12 years.
- *Tranexamic acid:* It can be used for heavy periods. It helps to reduce blood loss up to 50% during a period. It should not be used in women with history of thrombosis or convulsions.

Hormonal Treatments

Several medicines are available, making periods less painful, lighter, and more regular or stopping them altogether.

- *Norethisterone (NET):* This is a progesterone hormone tablet. To regulate periods and reduce blood loss it can be taken twice daily for 3 weeks, followed by a week off during which a period occurs. This can then be repeated for several months after which the tablets are stopped and periods monitored to see whether they have become lighter and more regular. Side effects include nausea, headache, and weight gain.
- *Combined hormonal contraceptive pill (CHC):* This is a tablet that contains two types of hormones—estrogen and progesterone. It works by stopping the ovaries producing an egg each month. The tablet is taken daily for 3 weeks and then during a 7-day break a light bleed occurs. It can be very helpful in the management of painful, heavy, and irregular periods. The CHC should not be used in women with history of focal migraine, who are overweight, have high blood pressure or heart disease.
- *Progesterone only pill—desogestrel:* Desogestrel is a newer type of pill that contains a progesterone hormone. It is a daily tablet taken without a break. In many women (over 50%), it may stop periods completely or there can be light bleeding.
- *Depo-Provera (Depo):* Depo is a long-acting progesterone hormone given as an injection every 10–12 weeks. The injection is usually given into the buttocks but can also be given in the thigh or upper arm. In many women (approximately 60%) the Depo will stop periods completely but in some women irregular, light bleeding, or troublesome bleeding can

occur. When it is stopped it can take up to 12 months for periods to return to normal. When it is regularly given every 12 weeks, it is over 99% effective as a contraceptive also.

CONCLUSION

Routine care is essential for the physical, mental, and emotional health of the adolescent with DS. The concerns and problems noted in this group are often the same as those seen in persons without DS. Helping to prepare parents and caregivers for this complex stage of life in DS is as important as counseling the normal adolescent.

SUGGESTED READING

1. Bovicelli L, Orsini LF, Rizzo N, Montacuti V, Bacchetta M. Reproduction in Down syndrome. Obstet Gynecol. 1982;59(6 Suppl):13S-7S.
2. Grinspon RP, Bedecarrás P, Ballerini MG, Iñiguez G, Rocha A, Mantovani Rodrigues Resende EA, et al. Early onset of primary hypogonadism revealed by serum anti-Müllerian hormone determination during infancy and childhood in trisomy 21. Int J Androl. 2011;34(5 Pt 2):e487-98.
3. Parizot E, Dard R, Janel N, Vialard F. Down syndrome and infertility: what support should we provide?. J Assist Reprod Genet. 2019;36(6):1063-7.
4. Whooten R, Schmitt J, Schwartz A. Endocrine manifestations of Down syndrome. Curr Opin Endocrinol Diabetes Obes. 2018;25(1):61-6.

CHAPTER 18

Neuropsychiatric and Behavior Disorders in Children with Down Syndrome

Krishnakumar P

INTRODUCTION

The general assumption that children with Down syndrome (DS) are happy, affectionate, and well behaved with an amiable disposition is not always true. Even though children with DS exhibit less behavior problems compared to children with nonspecific intellectual disability (ID) and those with other genetic syndromes such as Prader–Willi syndrome, they have more problems compared to typically developed children in the general population. Comorbid neuropsychiatric disorders are reported in 18–28% of children with DS with severe behavior problems in around 23% of children.

Behavior problems in children with DS are influenced by many factors such as age, gender, serotonin level, associated sleep problems, life stressors, hypothyroidism, medical illnesses, obesity, experience of abuse, and conditions causing physical pain. Children with mosaic DS are reported to have less behavior problems compared to children with pure trisomy 21. Family history of psychiatric disorders often predisposes to behavior disorders in children with DS. Externalizing behaviors such as aggression, hyperactivity, impulsivity, temper tantrums, and stubbornness are more common in young children with DS compared to adolescents and adults. Adolescents and adults are more likely to exhibit internalizing problems such as withdrawn behavior, features of depression, and anxiety. Some studies had reported more neuropsychiatric and behavior disorders in males compared to females with DS, but the data is insufficient to reach a conclusion.

Neurobiological changes associated with the presence of the extrachromosome may be predisposing to behavior disorders in children with DS. Both imaging studies and postmortem studies have demonstrated anatomical changes such as reduction in brain volume especially of the prefrontal cortex, hippocampus, and the cerebellum (structures involved in speech, language, memory, and executive functions). Impairments in functioning of the neurotransmitters such as gamma-aminobutyric acid (GABA), norepinephrine, glutamine, and *N*-methyl-D-aspartate (NMDA) as well as mitochondrial dysfunction and increased oxidative stress and micro-RNA abnormalities were reported in children with DS. Epigenetic changes such as histone modification and DNA methylation may also be contributing to the functional defects in DS.

NEURODEVELOPMENTAL DISORDERS

Attention Deficit Hyperactivity Disorder

Attention deficit hyperactivity disorder (ADHD) is the most common child psychiatric disorder in the general population, with a prevalence rate of 5–10% in children and adolescence. The three cardinal clinical features of ADHD are (1) hyperactivity, (2) impulsivity, and (3) inattention. There are three subtypes of ADHD—(1) predominantly hyperactive-impulsive type, (2) predominantly inattentive type, and (3) the combined type. The combined type is the most common type of ADHD in the general child population. As age advances, hyperactivity tends to decrease, and attention problems become more prominent.

Diagnosis of ADHD is based on clinical characteristics and there are no specific diagnostic tests. Diagnosis of ADHD is made only when the symptoms persist for >6 months and in two or more settings (e.g., school and home). The symptoms must begin before the age of 12 years and should not be secondary to other medical or psychological disorders and should cause impairment in social, academic, or occupational functioning. Comorbid psychiatric disorders such as oppositional defiant disorder, conduct disorder (CD), learning disorder, anxiety disorders, and depression are common in children with ADHD. Tics disorder and seizure disorder may coexist.

Drugs effective in controlling the symptoms of ADHD include stimulant drugs and nonstimulant drugs. Methylphenidate, dextroamphetamine, and their combinations are stimulant drugs while atomoxetine, clonidine belong to the nonstimulant group. For optimum results, pharmacotherapy should be combined with psychosocial interventions which include behavior therapy, attention enhancing tasks, dietary modifications along with school, and family-based interventions. Deficiency of micronutrients such as iron and zinc can cause attention problems and worsen hyperactivity and hence supplementation and appropriate dietary advice should be given if required. Children and parents should be advised regarding the importance of adequate sleep, rest, play, and regulating screen time.

Attention Deficit Hyperactivity Disorder in Children with Down Syndrome

The prevalence of ADHD in children with DS is higher than that in the general child population and the reported prevalence varies widely from 14 to 44%. Attention problems, hyperactivity and defects in executive functions are common in children with DS and may result in delayed diagnosis of ADHD. Diagnosis of ADHD is also difficult in children with DS and significant ID and communication problems. Even though the combined type is the most common type of ADHD in general population, in children with DS, inattention type of ADHD is reported to be more common. Higher rates of sleep disorders and disruptive behavior disorders are reported to occur in children with DS and ADHD.

Hearing and visual defects, anemia, sleep disorders, and thyroid disorders are common in children with DS. These are problems that can cause inattention and behavior issues and should be considered before making the diagnosis of ADHD. Cardiac status should be assessed before prescribing drug therapy for children with ADHD and DS since both stimulant and nonstimulant drugs are known to cause cardiac side effects.

Autism Spectrum Disorder

Autism spectrum disorder (ASD) is characterized by impairment in reciprocal social interaction and communication along with restricted repetitive and stereotyped patterns of behavior. The onset of the symptoms should be during the early developmental period. Defects in social interaction is manifested as impairment in the use of nonverbal behaviors (such as eye to eye contact, facial expressions, body postures, and gestures) and failure to develop age-appropriate peer relationships, inability to share enjoyment, interest or achievements with others, and lack of social or emotional reciprocity. Impairment in communication is manifested as delay or total lack of development of spoken language, impairment in the ability to initiate and sustain conversation, and stereotyped or repetitive use of language. The behavior pattern is often ritualistic and stereotyped. Stereotyped and repetitive motor mannerisms such as body twisting, hand or finger flapping or twisting, and inflexible adherence to routines or rituals may be present. There may be associated features such as abnormal fears and phobias, hyperactivity, eating and sleep problems, temper tantrums, aggressive behavior, and self-injurious behavior such as wrist biting. Seizures occur in about 25% of children. Even though children with ASD can have normal or above normal intelligence, most of them have varying degrees of ID.

Autism Spectrum Disorder in Children with Down Syndrome

The prevalence of ASD in children with DS is higher than that in the general population, regardless of the traditional description of children with DS as friendly and sociable. Earlier studies had reported lower prevalence rates, but recent studies report higher prevalence rates and vary from 5 to 12%. Some studies had reported prevalence rates as high as 41%. Severity of ASD increases with severity of ID. Communication problems and ID make early identification of ASD difficult, and the diagnosis is often delayed as late as 6–16 years. On the other hand, children with only DS may exhibit language stereotypes, ritualistic behavior, and strange likes and dislikes leading to overdiagnosis. It is recommended that specific rating scales should be used in children with DS to diagnose ASD.

DISRUPTIVE, IMPULSE CONTROL, AND CONDUCT DISORDERS IN CHILDREN WITH DOWN SYNDROME

Disruptive, impulse control, and CDs include oppositional defiant disorder, CD, and intermittent explosive disorder. These are disorders, characterized by problems in self-control of emotions and impulses that can lead to conflicts with law or social norms.

Oppositional Defiant Disorder

Oppositional defiant disorder (ODD) is characterized by irritable or angry mood, argumentative or defiant behavior, and vindictive nature. ODD is more common in boys and usually begins in the preadolescent age group. Children with ODD are often angry or irritable and lose their temper easily. They are often touchy, easily annoyed and argue frequently with peers, and figures of authority and are reluctant to comply with rules and regulations. ODD may precede childhood-onset type of CD or may be a milder type of CD.

Conduct Disorder

Behavior characteristics of CD in the general population include aggression toward people and animals, destruction of property, deceitfulness or theft, and serious violation of rules. Tendency toward aggression toward people and animals results in behaviors like bullying or threatening others, initiating physical fights with others, using weapons to harm others, forced sexual activity, and cruelty to animals. The tendency to destroy property is manifested as deliberate fire setting with the intention of causing damage and deliberate destroying property belonging to others. Deceitfulness or theft includes lying and stealing, cheating others like "con man." Children with CD may present with history of behaviors such as truancy (deliberately staying away from school and wandering outside), running away from home, or staying away from home without parental consent. Various types of delinquent behaviors and substance abuse may be associated with CD. CD can be childhood-onset type, adolescent-onset type, and unspecified-onset type. Symptoms begin to manifest before the age of 10 years in childhood onset CD while they occur during adolescence in the adolescent-onset type.

Children with DS: The prevalence of ODD and CD in children with DS is reported to be in the range of 10–15% and the prevalence is lower compared to children with nonspecific ID. The clinical presentation may vary with the age of the child and the severity of ID.

PSYCHOLOGICAL DISORDERS

Depression, anxiety disorders, and obsessive-compulsive disorders occur in individuals with DS usually during adolescence and adulthood and these internalizing disorders are not common in children. The prevalence of depression in individuals with DS is reported to be around 11%. Cognitive impairment and communication problems make the diagnosis of depression difficult in both children and adults with DS. Common symptoms of depression in individuals with DS include loss of interest, withdrawn behavior, loss of appetite, and sleep disturbance. Other classical symptoms of depression such as sad mood, crying spells, irritability, and aggressive behavior may also be present. ID and communication problems may mask the clinical presentation of depression and behavior change may be the presenting symptom. Depression should be considered in any child with ID if behavior problems that were not present previously occur.

Anxiety symptoms such as unreasonable fears, phobias, and somatic symptoms such as palpitation and tremors are reported in individuals with DS but the data on the prevalence of anxiety disorders in inconclusive.

Obsessive compulsive disorder (OCD) is characterized by obsessions and compulsions which are time consuming and cause significant distress or functional impairment. Obsessions are recurrent and persistent, unwanted, intrusive thoughts, urges, or images experienced by the individual and compulsions are repetitive behaviors or mental acts that the individuals are driven to perform with the aim of reducing the distress or anxiety. The prevalence of OCD in individuals with DS is 0.8–4.5% and is comparable to that in the general population. The clinical presentation of psychiatric symptoms may vary in individuals with DS depending on the degree of ID, communication problems, and other behavior characteristics. This fact should be considered, and appropriate and relevant rating scales should be used before making the diagnosis.

CONCLUSION

Contrary to the popular belief, neuropsychiatric and behavior disorders are not uncommon in individuals with DS. Externalizing behaviors occur predominantly in children with DS while internalizing behaviors tend to occur during adolescence and adulthood. ID and communication problems cause difficulty in identification of neuropsychiatric and behavior disorders in individuals with DS and the diagnosis is often delayed. Undiagnosed and untreated neuropsychiatric disorders can worsen the functioning of individuals with DS. Detailed clinical history and behavior observations, along with specific rating scales will help in early identification.

SUGGESTED READING

1. American Psychiatric Association. Diagnostic and Statistical Manual of Mental Disorders, 5th edition. Arlington, VA: American Psychiatric Association; 2013.

2. Ayano G, Demelash S, Gizachew Y, Tsegay L, Alati R. The global prevalence of attention deficit hyperactivity disorder in children and adolescents: An umbrella review of meta-analyses. J Affect Disord. 2023;339:860-6.
3. Baburamani AA, Patkee PA, Arichi T, Rutherford MA. New approaches to studying early brain development in Down syndrome. Dev Med Child Neurol. 2019;61(8):867-79.
4. DiGuiseppi C, Hepburn S, Davis JM, Fidler DJ, Hartway S, Lee NR, et al. Screening for autism spectrum disorders in children with Down syndrome: population prevalence and screening test characteristics. J Dev Behav Pediatr. 2010; 31(3):181-91.
5. Diniz NLF, Parlato-Oliveira E, Pimenta PGA, Araújo LA, Valadares ER. Autism and Down syndrome: early identification and diagnosis. Arq Neuropsiquiatr. 2022; 80(6):620-30.
6. Dykens EM, Kasari C. Maladaptive behavior in children with Prader–Willi syndrome, Down syndrome, and nonspecific mental retardation. Am J Ment Retard. 1997;102(3):228-37.
7. Dykens EM. Psychiatric and behavioral disorders in persons with Down syndrome. Ment Retard Dev Disabil Res Rev. 2007;13(3):272-8.
8. Ekstein S, Glick B, Weill M, Kay B, Berger I. Down syndrome and attention-deficit/hyperactivity disorder (ADHD). J Child Neurol. 2011;26(10):1290-5.
9. Ersoy SA, Güler HA, Çetin FH. Psychopathology in Down Syndrome. In: Dey S (Ed). Advances in Research on Down Syndrome. In Tech; 2018.
10. Esbensen AJ, Vincent LB, Epstein JN, Kamimura-Nishimura K, Wiley S, Angkustsiri K, et al. Co-occurring medical and behavioural conditions in children with Down syndrome with or without ADHD symptom presentation. J Intellect Disabil Res. 2022;66(3):282-96.
11. Gibbs MV, Thorpe JG. Personality stereotype of non-institutionalized Down syndrome children. Am J Ment Defic. 1983; 87(6):601-5.
12. Klein JA, Haydar TF. Neurodevelopment in Down syndrome: Concordance in humans and models. Front Cell Neurosci. 2022; 16:941855.
13. Reilly C. Autism spectrum disorders in Down syndrome: a review. Res Autism Spectr Disord. 2009;3:829-39.
14. Vacca RA, Bawari S, Valenti D, Tewari D, Nabavi SF, Shirooie S, et al. Down syndrome: Neurobiological alterations and therapeutic targets. Neurosci Biobehav Rev. 2019;98:234-55.
15. Vicari S, Pontillo M, Armando M. Neurodevelopmental and psychiatric issues in Down's syndrome: assessment and intervention. Psychiatr Genet. 2013;23(3):95-107.
16. Whittle N, Sartori SB, Dierssen M, Lubec G, Singewald N. Fetal Down syndrome brains exhibit aberrant levels of neurotransmitters critical for normal brain development. Pediatrics. 2007;120(6):e1465-71.
17. Zhang Y, Yang J, Jiang W, Li R, Zhu M, Xiong F, et al. Brain Development Measured With MRI in Children With Down Syndrome Correlates With Blood Biochemical Biomarkers. Pediatr Neurol. 2019;92:43-7.

SECTION

3 Developmental Therapies

CHAPTER 19

Early Intervention in Children with Down Syndrome

Muhlisa V

INTRODUCTION

Children with Down syndrome (DS) are expected to experience delays in different spheres of development. Early intervention is an essential part of helping children with DS to reach their maximum potential and sets the foundation for their overall development and future success. Early intervention services are designed to meet developmental needs of children from birth to 3 years of age, who have a delay in physical, cognitive, communicative, social, emotional, or adaptive development or have a diagnosed condition which has high probability of resulting in developmental delay. In this chapter, we look at why early intervention is so important, the key principles behind effective interventions, and the variety of interventions available to help children with DS and their families.

WHY EARLY INTERVENTION?

Early intervention and rehabilitation play a crucial role in improving the outcomes and quality of life for individuals with DS. Timely and tailored interventions during the early developmental stages can have far-reaching positive impacts on their physical, cognitive, communication, social, and emotional abilities.

- *To identify developmental delay early:* Early intervention helps to identify developmental delay and provides targeted interventions as soon as they are recognized. This prevents the widening of developmental gaps and helps children catch up in various areas of development.
- *To utilize the critical period of brain development:* The early years of life, particularly from birth to age three, are a period of rapid brain development and neuroplasticity. During this time, the brain is highly receptive to learning and forming new connections. Early intervention takes advantage of this period of high neuroplasticity to help children with DS to acquire essential skills, such as motor skills, communication abilities, and social interactions, that are foundational for later learning, independence, and quality of life.
- *To enhance cognitive abilities:* Children with DS experience cognitive challenges. The appropriate interventions can stimulate cognitive growth and promote skills such as memory, problem-solving, and logical thinking and prevent cognitive disabilities.
- *To improve communication skills:* Communication is a fundamental aspect of human interaction and learning. Early intervention focuses on improving communication skills, both verbal and nonverbal, enabling individuals with DS to better express themselves and engage with others.
- *To promote independence:* The rehabilitation interventions target motor skills, adaptive skills, and self-care abilities. These interventions empower individuals with DS to become more independent in daily activities and tasks.
- *To build social competence:* Early intervention supports the development of social skills, helping individuals with DS form meaningful relationships, engages in social interactions, and understands social cue.
- *To minimize behavioral challenges:* Early intervention can help address behavioral challenges by teaching appropriate coping strategies, communication methods, and emotional regulation techniques. This contributes to improved behavior and overall well-being.
- *To incorporate family involvement:* Early intervention programs engage families as active participants. Parents and caregivers receive guidance, training, and resources to support their child's development at home. The family-centered approach strengthens the child's support network.
- *To reduce financial burden:* Early intervention can lead to long-term cost savings by reducing the need for more intensive interventions or specialized services later in

life. It also increases the potential for individuals with DS to contribute to society in meaningful ways.

- *To promote inclusivity:* Early intervention and rehabilitation help to change the attitude of society toward individuals with DS as they develop skills and participate in various activities. It instils a sense of achievement, confidence, and self-esteem in individuals with DS, enabling them to pursue their interests and aspirations and thus promote inclusivity.

MULTIDISCIPLINARY TEAM

The multidisciplinary team collaborates to develop a comprehensive intervention plan that targets various aspects of the child's development. Regular communication, information sharing, and joint decision-making are essential for the success of the intervention. This collaborative approach recognizes that addressing the complex needs of children with DS requires expertise from various fields working together towards a common goal. The goals are set as short-term, intermediate, and long-term goals. The team members perform periodic reassessment of the child thus, improving the child's developmental outcomes and overall quality of life.

- *Pediatrician:* A medical professional plays a key role in the team by diagnosing DS, monitoring the child's health and growth, addressing medical concerns, and coordinating medical care.
- *Early intervention specialist or pediatric rehab physician:* This professional assesses the child's overall development and creates an individualized intervention plan. They coordinate the team, set goals, and ensure that the child's progress is monitored and tracked.
- *Speech-language pathologist (SLP):* An SLP focuses on improving the child's communication skills, speech articulation, language comprehension, and expressive language. They may introduce augmentative and alternative communication methods as needed.
- *Physical therapist (PT):* A PT assists with improving the child's motor skills, balance, coordination, and mobility. They may provide exercises, strategies, and activities to help the child develop physical abilities.
- *Occupational therapist (OT):* An OT helps the child develop fine motor skills, sensory integration, and the ability to perform activities of daily living (ADL). They address issues related to hand-eye coordination, grasping, and self-care skills.
- *Special educator:* A special educator focuses on providing tailored educational strategies to support the child's cognitive and academic development. They adapt teaching methods to the child's learning style and pace.
- *Behavioral therapist/psychologist:* They help to address behavioral challenges that might arise due to developmental delays. They provide strategies for managing behavior and promoting positive interactions.
- *Social worker:* They offer support to the child and family by addressing emotional and social needs. They provide counseling, coping strategies, and guidance for navigating social challenges.
- *Nutritionist or dietitian:* A nutrition expert ensures that the child is receiving appropriate dietary support for their growth and development. They might address any feeding difficulties that the child may have.
- *Parent/caregiver:* Parents and caregivers are vital members of the multidisciplinary team. Their insights, observations, and active participation contribute to the child's progress. They also learn techniques to support their child's development at home.

DEVELOPMENTAL ASSESSMENT AND INTERVENTION IN CHILDREN WITH DOWN SYNDROME

Children with DS usually follow same developmental sequence as typically developing children but they have quantitative and qualitative delays in various domains of development. They need to have regular developmental assessments in all developmental stages. The assessment provides information about child's abilities and framework to plan appropriate interventions and measure the progress. The assessments are done mainly in domains of motor, cognition, communication, social skills, and adaptive/self-help.

MOTOR DOMAIN

The motor skills are the abilities which help the child to manipulate, move around, and explore the environment around them. The components of motor function include postural control, gross motor skills, fine motor skills, reflexes and reactions, and sensory processing. The gross motor skill development refers to the use of large muscle groups of the body such as neck, trunk, and limbs for head control, sitting, standing, and walking **(Table 1)**.

TABLE 1: Gross motor development.

	Children with DS		***Typically developing children***	
Milestone	***Average age (months)***	***Range (months)***	***Average age (months)***	***Range (months)***
Head holding	5	3–5	3	1–4
Rolls over	8	4–12	5	2–10
Sits alone	9	6–16	7	5–9
Stands alone	18	12–38	11	9–16
Walks alone	23	13–48	12	9–17

Source: Cunningham C. Understanding Down Syndrome: An Introduction for Parents. Cambridge, MA: Brookline Books, 1996. pp. 185-91.

TABLE 2: Fine motor development.

	Children with DS		***Typically developing children***	
Milestone	***Average age (months)***	***Range (months)***	***Average age (months)***	***Range (months)***
Reaches out	6	4–11	4	2–6
Passes objects hand to hand	8	6–12	5.5	4–8
Builds tower of two cubes	30	14–32	15	10–19
Copies a circle	48	36–60	30	24–40

The fine motor skill development refers to the use of small muscles for manipulating objects with hand **(Table 2)**. The hands of children with DS differ with respect to the size, hypermobility of joints, hypotonia of muscles which affects the grasp strength, prehension, and dexterity. The developmental motor assessments are conducted using standardized tools such as Alberta Infant Motor Scale, Bayley Scales of Infant Development III, Peabody Developmental Motos Scales, Wee FIM, and Pediatric Evaluation of Disability Inventory. The assessment of motor control comprises of muscle tone and strength, control of movement, and posture. The children with DS have muscle hypotonia, hyperflexibility of joints, poor integration of proprioceptive, and the joint kinesthetic sense and have delay in the appearance and fading of reflexes and automatic patterns of movement. They are at risk for atlantoaxial subluxation due to the laxity of ligaments of the first two cervical vertebra. The prevalence of atlantoaxial subluxation is 4–8%.

The interventions for motor development are initiated in the first month for the development of postural control of neck and trunk muscles which facilitate future development of motor skills and prevent compensatory patterns and deformities secondary to constant atypical postures. The parents and family are educated about the proper positioning, handling, and therapeutic interventions. Physical therapy helps to improve the gross motor skills posture control, balance, and coordination required for ambulation. Occupational therapy helps to improve the fine motor skills which are important for the self-adaptive skills.

Development of postural control for head and upper trunk righting and upper extremity weight bearing in prone position, then ability to move against gravity to bring hands to midline and hands to mouth, proper alignment in sitting, scapular stability and upper extremity strength for fine motor control, movements in lower limbs to support standing, and development of transitional movements such as rolling, pivoting prone, crawling, coming up to sitting from supine, and sit to stand. Strength training is provided through resistive activities by promoting play with developmentally appropriate toys of varying weights such as lifting, pushing, and pulling toys. The balance and coordination training are very important for the coordinated control of trunk muscles, hips, knees, ankles, and feet to promote ambulation of children. Gait training is provided to improve the gait pattern. Fine motor skills training includes improving the prehension, grip and grasp strength, finger and thumb control, in hand manipulation, eye hand coordination, hand writing skills, and manipulation of self-adaptive devices.

TABLE 3: Communication skill development.

Milestone	Children with DS		Typically developing children	
	Average age (months)	Range (months)	Average age (months)	Range (months)
Responds to sounds	1	0.5–1.5	0	0–1
Babbles	7	4–8	4	2–6
Responds to simple instructions	9	6–16	7	5–9
First words spoken with meaning	18	13–36	14	10–23
Two-word phrases	30	18–60	20	15–30

COMMUNICATION DOMAIN

Communication is the process of exchange of information with each other. It includes verbal communication where spoken language is used to communicate and nonverbal communication where the facial expressions, pointing, and gestures are used to communicate **(Table 3)**. The speech and language domain of children with DS is significantly affected due to anatomical factors, hearing deficits, and cognitive factors. Hearing is the most important component of verbal language development. Neonatal hearing screening is conducted in all children using OAE (otoacoustic emission) followed by BERA (brainstem evoked response audiometry). They have high chance for conductive hearing loss due to high incidence of middle ear pathology like otitis media with effusion. The children with middle ear pathology require periodic monitoring of hearing under the supervision of an Otorhinolaryngologist.

Communication disorders in children are classified as hearing disorder, language disorder, and speech disorder. Hearing disorder results from an impaired sensitivity of auditory system. It includes difficulty in detecting, recognizing, discriminating, and comprehending auditory information. Language disorder involves the impairment of comprehension and or use of spoken, written, or other symbol systems. They are of three types of language disorder namely receptive language disorder, expressive language disorder and mixed receptive, and expressive language disorders. Speech disorder involves the impairment of production of speech sounds, fluency, and voice.

A SLP performs comprehensive assessment using standardized tool to evaluate the child's speech and language abilities and identifies the areas of strength and areas requiring training. Treatment plan is made based on the assessment and goal setting is done accordingly such as improving oral sensorimotor function, improving speech clarity and intelligibility, expanding vocabulary, improving language comprehension and expression, improving sentence structure, and improving social communication like understanding social cues, maintaining eye contact, taking turns in conversations and understanding nonverbal communication, and improving voice quality and fluency. Alternative augmentative communication (AAC) systems such as communication boards and picture exchange systems. And speech generating devices are beneficial for some children with DS. The parents and caregivers are trained to participate actively in the therapeutic interventions and reinforce communication goals at home. The child is reassessed in regular intervals to monitor the progress. Speech and language rehabilitation is a continuous process which evolves with child's requirement and developmentally appropriate goals for effective communication in daily life.

COGNITIVE DOMAIN

Cognition is the process of brain which allow us to think, remember, perform, and feel the emotions. The cognitive process components relevant with respect to DS are attention, learning, memory, reasoning, and problem solving. They have slower rate of cognitive development. The cognitive assessment is done using standardized test and represented as developmental quotient (DQ), intelligence quotient (IQ), mental age (MA), and age equivalent (AE). The incidence of autism in children with DS is about 15% and attention deficit hyperactivity disorder (ADHD) is 6–8%. The regular behavior monitoring of children with DS in the toddler and preschool age is very important. Clinical psychologist or behavioral therapist in the multidisciplinary team will address this issue.

The cognitive domain of development overlaps with all other developmental domains. Children with DS are likely to have mild-to-moderate cognitive delay. The cognitive skills are trained using the principles of learning theory. Rehabilitation interventions for cognitive development focus on improving cognitive functioning, promote learning, and improve problem solving and adaptive skills. The child is provided with activities for his chronological age and developmental age to stimulate their cognitive abilities. The interventions are initiated at an early age. The interventions are provided in different environments like home, center based, day care, and social gatherings using different modalities such as objects, pictures, sound and light by different persons, parents, therapists, and teachers. Interventions to improve attention and concentration are important as they are essential for learning and daily tasks. Memory enhancing intervention and strategies to improve short-term and long-term memory are needed. The children should be provided with opportunities with other children in structured and semistructured activities like group learning experience. They should be provided with opportunities for generalization and exploration. Cognitive tools and strategies such as visual schedules, check lists, and structured routine help to improve cognitive functioning and independence in daily life. Behavioral and emotional issues are present in some children. The parental and caregiver training are an integral part in rehabilitation. They are provided training and guidance on how to monitor behavior, reinforce cognitive interventions, and strategies at home. The child is reassessed in regular intervals with standardized tools to ensure progress and optimization of therapeutic interventions. Cognitive rehabilitation is a continuous process which focuses on enhancing the cognitive potential and achieves greater independence in their daily lives.

SOCIAL DOMAIN

Social development is the process through which the children learn to build relationships. Social skills are a set of abilities that initiate and maintain positive social relationships, develop friendships with peers, and create adjustments in future life. Social skill development is very important. The social functioning of children with DS is relatively less delayed than other areas of development. The children with DS develop good social skills and appropriate behavior with proper training and guidance. Social skill deficits can lead to difficulties namely externalizing problems such as maladaptive behavior, antisocial behavior, and internalizing problems like lack of confidence, anxiety, and depression.

The assessment of social development depends on other developmental domain skill acquisition such as cognitive skills, communication skills, hearing status, gross motor, and fine motor skills.

- Social initiation—the ability to begin interactions like showing or giving objects to others for social purposes
- Social imitation—imitating actions of others
- Age expected reciprocity like turn taking during play
- Child's attachment behavior pattern toward caregiver/ parent like neutrality, excessive clinging, or avoidance
- Social interaction with familiar and unfamiliar adults and peers
- Child's ability to make transition from one play activity or toy to another
- Joint attention—behavior in which two people focus on an object or event for the purpose of interacting with each other. It involves using gestures, eye contact, or other forms of communication to share the experience of an object or event along with another person
- Direct observation of child's interaction with parents, caregivers, siblings, and other children
- The assessment of home environment such as nurturing, stimulation, cultural values, social rules, and customs in the family

The children with DS are exposed to different social situations to stimulate and selectively reinforce the appropriate behaviors, to improve peer interactions, to promote generalization, to facilitate communication and language development. Child's attention in activities is requested and positively reinforced with appropriate responses. Child's play skills are facilitated by allowing them to interact with children in cooperative play. In cooperative play, the cooperation and team work help to improve critical social skills like turn taking, sharing, and problem solving. Role playing in social situations like greeting in conversation helps children with DS to practice social skills in a safe and supportive environment. Group therapy along with individual therapy improves social skills in these children.

SELF HELP/ADAPTIVE SKILLS

The self-help skills or adaptive skills also known as functional skills/ADL. It is an important skill the children with DS need to attain for overall quality of life of the children and their caregivers. One of the primary aims in the rehabilitation of these children is to attain age appropriate self-help skills **(Table 4)**. The deficits in other domain may affect the self-help skill attainment such as deficit in body awareness, difficulty in maintaining attention, delay in motor skill development, and motor planning deficit.

Children with DS need more repetitions, consistency, and modifications to facilitate independence. For feeding training, they require consistency in meal time, premeal routines, proper positioning and posture, and modified feeding utensils such as spoon with thick handle and cup with two handles. Children are usually independent in removing clothes before they are independent in putting on clothes. The modifications such as fastener-free clothing until child learns appropriate fine motor skills such as zipping and buttoning, Velcro instead of buttons, zippers and attaching easy to grip zipper pulls. The toilet training is initiated when child's motor skills and cognitive development are adequately achieved. The regularity in elimination is an indication of bowel and bladder control. The child has to be familiar with the training environment. The consistency in using the same washroom is better. The process of developing adaptive/self-help skills should be continuous, integrated into all activities by family members, and professionals throughout the intervention and everyday activities.

TABLE 4: Social and self-adaptive development.

	Children with DS		***Typically developing children***	
Milestone	***Average age (months)***	***Range (months)***	***Average age (months)***	***Range (months)***
Responsive smile	2	1.5–4	1	1–2
Plays peek-a-boo	11	9–16	8	5–13
Drinks from cup	20	12–30	12	9–17
Bowel control	36	20–60	24	16–48
Dresses self (unassisted)	3.5–8.5 years			3.25–5 years

TABLE 5: Age-specific interventions.

Age	***Communication domain***	***Cognitive domain***	***Motor domain***
0–4 months	• Facilitation of oromotor functioning and feeding • Stimulation techniques • Tracking auditory stimulation • Orienting to voices • Vocalizing when spoken to	• Visual tracking • Name calling • Reading and singing to child regularly	• To prevent compensatory movement pattern which interfere with subsequent motor development • To prevent deformities secondary to persistent atypical postures • Development of postural control, control of head and trunk
4–12 months	• Encourage babbling • Use of informal gestures like pointing • Language stimulation techniques and activities appropriate for individual child • Monitor oromotor function—strength, coordination of lip, jaw, and tongue function	Continue teaching of cognitive skills	*Gross motor skills:* • Development of postural control for head and trunk, righting and upper extremity weight bearing in prone • Development of sufficient head and trunk control for proper alignment in sitting • Development of postural control, scapular stability, and upper extremity strength for fine motor control • Development of transitional movements such as rolling, pivoting, belly crawls, getting in and out of sitting • Development of ability to move against gravity to bring hands to mid line and hands to mouth *Fine motor skill:* • Training initiated at 6 months • Eye hand coordination • Grasp and grip strengthening • Transfer of objects from hand

Contd...

Contd...

Age	Communication domain	Cognitive domain	Motor domain
12–24 months	• Speech and language interventions according to child's need • Focus on parent training for language stimulation • Provide opportunity for interaction with other children through play group/day care/ group therapy • Continue oromotor function	• Continue age appropriate cognitive skills • Provide group learning experiences	*Gross motor skills:* • Focused on use of muscle control, posture, and movement rather than compensatory pattern • Development of creeping pattern on hands and knees • Development of postural control for translational movements such as supine to sitting and pull to stand • To improve balance and coordination of trunk muscles • Use of coordinated control in hips, knees, ankles, and feet *Fine motor skills:* • To improve prehension pattern • Grip strength • Finger and thumb control • Eye-hand coordination • In hand manipulation • Release of objects
24–36 months	• Continue speech and language intervention to improve receptive and expressive language skills • Improve vocabulary • Improve mean length of utterance • Improve speech intelligibility	• Interaction with children in structured and semi structured activities • Generalization and exploration	*Gross motor skills:* • Development of independent walking • Development of stair climbing • Development of high-level motor skills *Fine motor:* • Use of writing materials • Turning knobs and lids

Source: Vietze PM, Arvedson JC, Bogin D, Doret W, Hanin L, Harris C. Clinical Practice Guideline Report of the Recommendations Down Syndrome Assessment and Intervention for Young Children (age 0–3 years). New York: State Department of Health; 2006. pp. 162-6.

CONCLUSION

Early intervention acknowledges the critical role of the early years in shaping a child's development and recognizes that timely and appropriate support can lead to better outcomes and increased independence for children with developmental delays. It is crucial to approach each child with DS as an individual and provide them with tailored interventions that address their unique strengths and challenges **(Table 5)**. Early intervention and ongoing support play a vital role in helping individuals with DS reach their full potential and lead fulfilling lives.

SUGGESTED READING

1. Barbosa RT, de Oliveira AS, de Lima Antão JY, Crocetta TB, Guarnieri R, Antunes TP, et al. Augmentative and alternative communication in children with Down's syndrome: A systematic review. BMC Pediatrics. 2018;18:1-6.
2. Cardoso AC, Campos AC, Santos MM, Santos DC. Motor performance of children with down syndrome and typical development at 2 to 4 and 26 months. Pediatr Phys Ther. 2015;27(2):135-41.
3. Cicchetti D, Beeghly M. Children with Down Syndrome: A Developmental Perspective. United Kingdom: Cambridge University Press; 1990.
4. Cicchetti D, Ganiban J. The Organization and Coherence of Developmental Processes in Infants and Children with Down Syndrome. In: Hodapp RM, Burack JA, Zigler E (Eds). Issues in the Developmental Approach to Mental Retardation. United Kingdom: Cambridge University Press; 1990. pp. 169-225.
5. Cunningham C. Understanding Down Syndrome: An Introduction for Parents. Cambridge, MA: Brookline Books; 1996.
6. Girolametto LE. Improving the social-conversational skills of developmentally delayed children: an intervention study. J Speech Hearing Disord. 1988;53(2):156-67.
7. Grieco J, Pulsifer M, Seligsohn K, Skotko B, Schwartz A. Down syndrome: Cognitive and behavioral functioning across the lifespan. Am J Med Genet C Semin Med Genet. 2015;169(2):135-49.
8. Guralnick MJ. The effectiveness of early intervention for children with cognitive and general developmental delays. In: Guralnick MJ (Ed). The Effectiveness of Early Intervention for At-Risk and Handicapped Children. New York, NY: Academic Press; 1987.

9. Harris SR. Effects of neurodevelopmental therapy on motor performance of infants with Down's syndrome. Dev Med Child Neurol. 1981;23(4):477-83.
10. Hauser-Cram P, Warfield ME, Shonkoff JP, Krauss MW, Upshur CC, Sayer A. Family influences on adaptive development in young children with Down syndrome. Child Develop. 1999;70(4):979-89.
11. Hines S, Bennett F. Effectiveness of early intervention for children with Down syndrome. Mental Retardation Develop Disabil Res Rev. 1996;2(2):96-101.
12. Needham AW, Nelson EL, Short AD, Daunhauer lA, Fidler DJ. The Emergence of fine motor skills in children with Down syndrome. Hodapp RM, Fidler DJ (Eds). International Review of Research in Developmental Disabilities. United States: Academic Press; 2021;60:113-51.
13. Novak I, Morgan C. High-risk follow-up: early intervention and rehabilitation. Handbook of clinical neurology. 2019;162:483-510.
14. O'Toole C, Lee ASY, Gibbon FE, van Bysterveldt AK, Hart NJ. Parent-mediated interventions for promoting communication and language development in young children with Down syndrome. Cochrane Database Syst Rev. 2018;10(10):CD012089.
15. Patterson T, Rapsey CM, Glue P. Systematic review of cognitive development across childhood in Down syndrome: implications for treatment interventions. J Intellec Disabil Res. 2013;57(4):306-18.
16. Pueschel SM, Findley TW, Furia J, Gallagher PL, Scola FH, Pezzullo JC. Atlantoaxial instability in Down syndrome: roentgenographic, neurologic, and somatosensory evoked potential studies. J Pediatr. 1987;110(4):515-21.
17. Rast MM, Harris SR. Motor control in infants with Down syndrome. Developmental Med Child Neurol. 1985;27(5): 682-5.
18. Reilly C. Autism spectrum disorders in Down syndrome: A review. Res Autism Spect Dis. 2009;3(4):829-39.
19. Roberts JE, Price J, Malkin C. Language and communication development in Down syndrome. Ment Retard Dev Disabil Res Rev. 2007;13(1):26-35.
20. Seager E, Sampson S, Sin J, Pagnamenta E, Stojanovik V. A systematic review of speech, language and communication interventions for children with Down syndrome from 0 to 6 years. Int J Lang Commun Dis. 2022;57(2):441-63.
21. Soresi S, Nota L. A social skill training for persons with Down's syndrome. European psychologist. 2000;5(1):34.
22. Sroufe LA. Early relationships and the development of children. Infant Ment Health J. 2000;21(1-2):67-74.
23. Tedeschi AS, Roizen NJ, Taylor HG, Murray G, Curtis CA, Parikh AS. The prevalence of congenital hearing loss in neonates with Down syndrome. J Pediatr. 2015;166(1):168-71.
24. US Department of Education. (2005). To assure the free appropriate public education of all children with disabilities (Individuals with Disabilities Education Act, Section 618). Twenty-third Annual Report to Congress on the Implementation of the Individuals with Disabilities Education Act 2001. [online] Available from http://www.ed.gov/about/reports/annual/osep/2001/index.html [Last accessed April,2025].
25. Uyanik M, Bumin G, Kayihan HÜ. Comparison of different therapy approaches in children with Down syndrome. Pediatr Int. 2003;45(1):68-73.
26. Wang PP, Bellugi U. Williams syndrome, Down syndrome, and cognitive neuroscience. Am J Dis Child. 1993;147(11): 1246-51.

CHAPTER 20

Down Syndrome: A Psychological Perspective

KS Mohan, Sharada Mohan

"I have Down syndrome but that is not all I am."

—Sarah Gordy, British Actor.

INTRODUCTION

There are many features of Down syndrome (DS), but not all are seen in each case. Pathologically, the brain is small and there are widespread defects in the cortical cell layers and in the number of ganglion cells. Whole gyri may be faulty in development. The process apparently is stationary; regressive changes are not seen.

The personality development may be immature and emotional. Tantrums during childhood are frequent. In adult stage, most are happy, amicable with a tractable disposition, conscientious in work, and undemanding at home.

The neuropathological changes may not necessarily be accompanied by clinical symptoms of dementia until the fourth to fifth decade of life. Mentally, the subject is docile and tractable. The appearance will be of higher mental capacity than is really present because of imitativeness. A few are hyperactive and sometimes destructive. Subjects were noted for a deteriorating intellectual performance from middle age onward. However, the steady, if slow, neurological development means that educational programs which began from 6 months of age have been attended with significant success in terms of childhood achievements.

Whenever a child with DS presents at a primary care source, it can be challenging to the medical practitioner. The condition often requires the intervention of many specialists and professional as well as voluntary service agencies. Involvement of a clinical psychologist is one such which would play a crucial part in the evaluation and management of the child.

Usually, a case is referred by a medical professional to a psychologist to assess developmental skills and intellectual abilities. Basically, the areas covered are:

- *Socialization:* This includes behavior, appropriate for living and interacting with persons around. Unless a child receives attention for his/her behavior, there will be no motivation to learn new behavior, e.g., a child's cry gets mother's attention. Learning takes place in this way, and further changes in behavior occur with the approval and disapproval of the family.
- *Language:* Cognitive and socialization skills are closely linked to language development. A pattern of listening - understanding - expressing has to be established. It starts with attending and responding to the mother's voice. Gradually, sounds take on a meaning. The child responds with his own sound, and the family's reactions become reinforcements. The child has to be talked to (input) and encouraged to verbalize (output).
- *Self-help:* A child has to learn skills of direction such as eating, bathing, toilet care, and dressing. This makes him independent and also reduces the need for care and supervision by family.
- *Cognition:* This involves the development of concepts (e.g., similarities and differences), numbers, and such others. Remembering to act in certain ways in certain situations, all require cognitive skills and in turn influence other areas of development.
- *Motor development:* Co-ordinated movements of body muscles are necessary to express skills. The ability to maintain postures, balancing, and posturing is essential to explore and understand one's surroundings.

A child's intellectual level of development is assessed by a clinical psychologist based on one's developmental history and by administering the intelligence quotient (IQ) tests. One arrives at the IQ by arriving at a child's mental age (MA) on the tests and comparing it to the child's

TABLE 1: Intelligence quotient (IQ) scores.

IQ score	*Category*
90–110	Average intelligence
70–89	Slow learner
50–69	Mild retardation
35–49	Moderate retardation
20–34	Severe retardation
<20	Profound retardation

chronological age (CA). Hence, IQ = MA/CA × 100. The score, which is derived from this, helps to place a child in the categories which are shown in **Table 1**.

The results thus obtained give a profile of the child's assets and liabilities. This potential is used in various skills training programs, which must be tailor-made for each child. These programs are carried out at schools, clinics attached to hospitals, or institutions. Parents/caretakers are actively involved in these programs and they should benefit the child at home and in other social situations.

Behavioral Problems in Down Syndrome

All living organisms show variability in their behaviors. Behavioral problems are seen in all children. Some of the common problems likely to be encountered in children with DS are discussed briefly here:

- *Social skills:* Many children with DS are social and affectionate. Some are shy and have to be encouraged to make eye contact and greet people.
- *Communication skills:* Ability to express and verbalize one's needs and respond verbally to others' queries will require training.
- *Self-help skills:* Basic hygiene, toilet training, eating, dressing, and play skills will require constant supervision and guidance.
- *Attention deficits:* The children could have distractibility or short attention span. This could affect verbal short-term memory and explicit long-term memory. Overall, attention is important for any type of new learning.
- *Motivation:* To facilitate new learning, one has to be motivated. Hence, motivators or positive reinforcers are used to develop and maintain new behaviors. Negative reinforcers are used to fade out inappropriate behaviors.
- *Tantrums and aggression:* Usually, tantrums are a response to frustrations at not being able to convey what they want or being at a loss to do what others demand. Often these can be controlled with behavior therapy techniques. Only if the aggression is harmful to others or self-destructive in nature, medication should be used for initial control.
- *Anxieties and fears:* Like all children, kids with DS however have strong visual memories, hence they may replay fearful situations in their mind. In therapy, one has to identify and work to alleviate their fear. Extreme phobias and psychotic fears may require medication.

Behavior disorders may have to be treated with antipsychotics. It is found that doses are generally high to control the behavior. On the other hand, children in the community are relatively deprived of consistent and adequate pharmacotherapy that might facilitate their care.

It is important that associated physical health problems should be identified and treatment given as required. Hypothyroidism may be congenital or may develop later, the incidence increasing with age. It can negatively affect cognitive function and is preventable with thyroid hormone replacement.

The birth of a baby with DS is an upsetting experience for most parents. Mothers who fail to see their children frequently in the first days of life may fail to develop bonding or maternal love. Hence, early bonding to avoid rejection is essential. Encouragement and counseling of both the parents alone and together should be the responsibility of the counselor.

The quality of life and life expectancy have improved markedly owing to improved developmental care, availability of medicines, and surgical correction of anomalies, especially those affecting the heart.

Overall, the aim is to increase desirable behavior and reduce undesirable behavior. Hence, the psychologist's approach is that of behavior modification therapy. The guidelines would be to recognize the child's strengths. Use clear and simple language to communicate. Establish a routine and follow that to avoid confusion. Break each task to be taught into simple steps to facilitate early learning and avoid frustration. Use multisensory teaching methods. Do not teach too much at once, but one skill at a time. Only through extensive practice will the child become adept at the tasks. Periodic review of previously learned behavior is to be done and retraining for those which may have been forgotten.

No doubt, the training process is uphill and arduous. However, the successes, both big and small, are highly rewarding to the parents and child and give hopes of leading a more meaningful life.

CONCLUSION

While caring for a person with DS may come with challenges, it is often deeply rewarding. Individuals with DS each have unique personalities and strengths, and many respond well to therapy and support. With understanding, acceptance, and inclusion in family life and the broader community, what may initially seem daunting can evolve into a journey of growth and connection. A compassionate, supportive environment plays a vital role in enabling individuals with DS to lead fulfilling and meaningful lives.

SUGGESTED READING

1. Al-Biltagi M. Downs Syndrome Children - An Update. Bentham Books, 2015.
2. Aubitz A. The Many Faces of Down Syndrome: Stories of Inspiration, Hope and Laughter. Special Stars Publishing. 2016, pp. 142.
3. Burack JA, Edgin JO, Abbeduto L. The Oxford Handbook of Downs Syndrome and Development. Oxford Library of Psychology Series, 2023.
4. Chicoine B, McGuire D. Guide to Good Mental Health: For Teens & Adults with Downs Syndrome. Woodbine House Inc.,US, 2010.
5. Prasher V, Santos FH. Excelling in Life with Downs Syndrome. Nova Science Publishers, 2021, pp. 238.

CHAPTER 21

Enhancing Communication in Children with Down Syndrome: Recent Advances in Intervention

Neethu Koroth, Sreerenthu S Viswan, Fayeda TK, Rasitha Harish

INTRODUCTION

This chapter gives insights on speech and language issues in children with Down syndrome and about the speech and language intervention strategies that can be used. Language disturbances seen in children with Down syndrome include delayed receptive and expressive language skills. They typically have stronger receptive language skills than expressive language skills, with relative strengths in pragmatic skills, receptive vocabulary and narrative skills, particularly for events, themes, and story elements. Some children are found to be having impaired cognitive skills which makes it difficult to attain the speech and language milestones normally when compared to a typically developing child. Researchers also reported that children with Down syndrome show significant delays in phonological working memory, phonological processing, expressive vocabulary, microstructural narrative elements, and syntax, specifically with regard to expression of complex syntactical forms, grammatical morphemes, and negation. The natural environment with language stimulation might not be enough to stimulate the receptive and expressive language skills in children who have comorbid conditions, such as intellectual disability.

Apart from language skills, motor speech skills are also found to be affected in children with Down syndrome. Most of the children with Down syndrome have a complaint of limited verbal output along with impaired or reduced motor speech skills. Studies have reported that neuroanatomical deficiencies in these children may be related to delays in general motor and motor speech milestones.

The motor speech characteristics seen in children with Down syndrome include childhood dysarthria (CD), childhood apraxia of speech (CAS), or both. CD is a disorder of neuromuscular execution where speech disturbances such as speech sound distortions, slow, fast, or irregular rate, and abnormal pitch, loudness, resonance, or voice quality are seen. These disturbances occur as a result of neuromuscular problems which affects the tone, strength, range, timing, and coordination of the speech musculature. CAS is a disorder of motor planning and programming where speech issues, such as difficulty with sequencing articulatory movements, phonemes and syllables, trial and error groping behaviors, and inconsistent articulatory errors are seen. Shriberg et al. (2010) suggested that the term motor speech disorder-not otherwise specified (MSD-NOS) can be used when a child cannot be labeled as having CD or CAS.

Speech intelligibility is another major concern in these children. These issues persist into their adulthood and can hinder their communication abilities and social interactions. Speech intelligibility issues can be due to several factors such as disturbances in voice, articulation, resonance, fluency, and prosody. Even though craniofacial issues are accounted for speech intelligibility problems, all aspects of the speech problems are of various other factors also. Since hearing loss is also prevalent in children with Down syndrome and has a direct effect on their speech skills, it should also be periodically monitored.

Speech and Language Assessment

The speech and language evaluation begins with a detailed case history, and it includes the following:

- Demographic details
- Brief history and complaints
- Birth history
- Family history
- Medical history
- *Developmental milestones:* They include motor, speech and language, and sensory development.
- *Oral peripheral mechanism examination (OPME):* Assessment of the tone, strength, rate, and range of movement of articulators at rest and during speech
- Feeding skills

- Vegetative skills
- Prelinguistic skills
- Social skills
- Parent-child interaction
- Assessment of Linguistic skills using appropriate test materials such as the Receptive Expressive Emergent Language cale (REELS), and the three-dimensional language acquisition test (3-DLAT)
- Assessment of speech skills (articulation, voice, fluency, resonance, and respiration)

The case history commences with demographic details, which include the name, age/gender, and address, followed by a brief history which includes information about the speech and language issues faced by the child, its onset, and course. Detailed birth history, family history, and medical history are a part of the assessment. The speech language pathologist (SLP) performs the OPME to identify abnormal tone, strength, rate or range of movement of the articulators such as lips, tongue, hard palate, soft palate, jaw, and teeth. Assessment of feeding skills, vegetative skills, prelinguistic skills, and social skills is carried out thereafter. Parent-child interaction is an important factor which needs to be considered. Quantitatively and qualitatively better parent-child interaction helps in better linguistic skills. Poor interaction between the child and the parents often leads to a delay in receptive and expressive language skills.

A detailed assessment of the receptive and expressive language skills helps the SLP to identify the child's language age. Often, children with Down syndrome are found to have receptive and expressive language delay, but sometimes they are found to have expressive language delay only. Assessment of speech skills mainly includes test materials to assess articulatory skills, resonance, and overall speech intelligibility. Articulatory errors include distortions (mostly due to macroglossia), substitutions, additions, and omissions. These articulatory errors in turn affect the overall speech intelligibility.

SPEECH AND LANGUAGE THERAPY

After carrying out the speech and language assessment using appropriate test materials and protocols, the SLP sheds light on the intervention strategies and provides suitable recommendations. Multidisciplinary approach aids in better prognosis as different professionals—pediatrician, otorhinolaryngologists, physiotherapists, occupational therapists, audiologists, speech language pathologists, psychologists—engage in planning and executing the interventional strategies.

Why is Early Intervention Important?

Another important aspect that needs to be considered is "early intervention", which is a systematic program that is designed to address the developmental delays seen in children with Down syndrome or other disabilities. Early intervention begins shortly after birth and should usually continue until the child is eligible for kindergarten. An amendment to IDEA in 2004 allows states to have early intervention programs that may continue until the child enters, or is eligible to enter, kindergarten. The sooner the early intervention begins, the better, and it is never too late to start. Development is a continuous process that begins at conception and proceeds stage by stage in an orderly sequence. There are specific milestones in each of the four areas of development (gross and fine motor abilities, language skills, social development, and self-help skills) that serve as prerequisites for the stages that follow.

Speech and language therapy is a critical component of early intervention. Children with Down syndrome are often found to be late talkers. They tend to say their first words after 2 or 3 years of age. There are many skills that they must acquire before they learn to form words. These skills include ability to imitate and echo sounds, turn-taking skills (learned through games like "peek-a-boo"), visual skills (looking at the speaker and objects), auditory skills (listening to music, speech, or speech sounds for lengthening periods of time), tactile skills (learning about touch and exploring objects in the mouth), oral motor skills (using the tongue and moving the lips), and cognitive skills (understanding object permanence and cause-and-effect relationships). The SLP focuses on these skills during the intervention before or while working on the language abilities of the child. During the speech and language therapy, the SLP often works on improving the following skills, namely, prelinguistic skills, oro-motor skills, feeding skills, speech skills, and language skills.

PRELINGUISTIC SKILLS

Prelinguistic skills are the prerequisites for language development in children. Children with poor prelinguistic skills are observed to have delayed language skills. Prelinguistic skills such as the ability to imitate and echo, the ability to point out, name call response, attention, concentration, and eye contact are necessary. These will be worked upon in the speech and language therapy session using suitable play activities and games.

OROMOTOR SKILLS

An oromotor skill generally refers to the movement of the face and oral area, especially the movements related to speech. Children with Down syndrome often have difficulty with oromotor skills. Traditional oromotor exercises are being used during the intervention, and some of the goals worked upon are: To improve the strength, rate, and range of movement of articulators, such as lips, and tongue, and to reduce tongue thrust.

VEGETATIVE SKILLS AND FEEDING SKILLS

Other skills that will be worked upon are the vegetative skills and the feeding skills. Children with neuromuscular deficits often exhibit difficulties with vegetative skills—such as sucking, chewing, biting, straw drinking, etc.—and feeding skills. These skills are sometimes compromised as the acquisition of effective motor skills gets affected, and it leads to the development of potential feeding problems and swallowing dysfunction. Anil et al. (2019) conducted a study on children with Down syndrome in the age range of 2–7 years and reported that they were having difficulty with all three phases of swallow (oral, pharyngeal, and esophageal phases).

SPEECH SKILLS

Articulation and clarity of speech are often seen to be affected in children with Down syndrome. Children often have articulatory errors because of structural abnormalities such as macroglossia and high-arched palate. Articulation therapy focuses on improving the placement and manner of articulation by giving visual, tactile, and auditory feedback, as well as by using specific techniques.

Sounds are initially targeted in the isolation level, and it is followed by syllables, words, phrases, sentences, and conversation. Once the error sounds get corrected, it often leads to improved speech clarity. The SLP then works on improving the speech clarity in conversation level by making use of certain techniques, such as open-mouth approach.

LANGUAGE SKILLS

Speech and language therapy interventions aim to support the development of both receptive and expressive language skills, enhancing effective communication. Speech therapy activities usually include:

- *Providing visual aids:* Using visual aids such as flash cards and objects to build receptive and expressive vocabulary, and thereby helping the child to associate words with images. This enhances expressive vocabulary and communicative skills.
- *Play:* Play can be included in the form of role play, structured play, anticipatory games, etc., which aim to enhance the linguistic skills.

The frequency of the speech and language therapy depends on the severity of the language disorder. The duration of the session usually remains 45 minutes, and depending on the child's language level, sessions are allotted: Thrice a week, twice a week, or on a daily basis. During the therapy session, the SLP takes up skills that need to be worked upon and determines the specific goals, namely long-term and short-term goals. Then, through activities that target the short-term goals, the SLP works on the specific goals. Once the child achieves 80–85% consistency, the SLP takes up other short-term goals and works on that.

RECENT ADVANCES IN INTERVENTION STRATEGIES

Oral Placement Therapy

Currently, oral placement therapy (OPT) is considered an important addition to the traditional speech treatment methods for children with placement and movement deficits. OPT represents a paradigm of tactile-proprioceptive treatment method, which is used to improve articulator awareness, placement (dissociation, grading, and direction of movement), stability, and muscle memory; all of these are necessary for the development of speech clarity. The key feature of the definition of OPT lies in a child's ability/disability to imitate auditory-visual stimuli and follow instructions of verbal oral placements. The hierarchy of oral placement for speech clarity and feeding safety is as follows: Feeding – phonation – resonation – articulation. It is mentioned that a feeding program can be initiated prior to OPT for those with severe cognitive deficits. Likewise, supplemental activities can be incorporated for those who cannot achieve jaw or lip closure (which is generally associated with high muscle tone) before initiating articulation activities.

Oral placement therapy is a form of oral motor treatment done through exercises by focusing on the movement and coordination of the jaw, lips, tongue, and cheeks. It is often employed to support children with Down syndrome, who may experience challenges such as oral-motor coordination difficulties and low muscle tone (hypotonia).

Effectiveness of OPT for Individuals with Down Syndrome

Various researches and clinical observations suggest that OPT can be beneficial for children with Down syndrome, specifically in addressing challenges related to speech clarity, feeding, and overall oral motor function. These results may vary depending on the individual's needs and the expertise of the therapist. However, more systematic researches are still required to address all the areas and quantify the efficacy of OPT.

How does OPT help?

- *Improves speech clarity:* Down syndrome is often associated with challenges in speech, such as articulation difficulties and reduced intelligibility. OPT aims to strengthen the muscles required for speech, improving articulatory skills, and overall intelligibility.
- *Improves feeding skills:* Chewing and swallowing can be impaired due to low muscle tone (hypotonia). OPT helps in improving coordinated oral motor movements and thereby improving feeding skills. Many goals such as tongue lateralization and retraction, lip closure, jaw stability, jaw symmetry, jaw grading, and independent feeding can be addressed while working on feeding; hence, feeding is important to an OPT program.
- *Improves jaw stability:* Many with Down syndrome experience issues with jaw stability, which can impact both speech and feeding. Exercises targeting the symmetrical/asymmetrical jaw weakness enhance the articulation and feeding skills.
- *Addresses sensory-motor integration:* OPT can help individuals to process sensory information more effectively, which is observed to be beneficial for those with oral hypersensitivity or low sensitivity.

Limitations

- *Limited high-quality evidence:* Though many practitioners report positive outcomes, there is a lack of robust, peer-reviewed research proving the efficacy of OPT, especially in comparison to other therapeutic approaches.
- *Requires skilled implementation:* Success rates with OPT depend heavily on the therapist's expertise and the customization of exercises to address the individual's specific needs.
- *Variations in the outcome:* The results of OPT can vary significantly from individual to individual, with some showing marked improvement and others experiencing limited benefits. OPT is often most effective when used in conjunction with traditional speech-language therapy.

While OPT has shown a promising effect for children with Down syndrome in improving oral motor skills, its effectiveness needs to be assessed on a case-by-case basis. More systematic research is still needed to establish its long-term benefits and efficacy in treating various oral placement disorders. Families considering OPT should consult with experienced professionals and consider a holistic approach to intervention.

CONCLUSION

Children with Down Syndrome have many speech and language difficulties, it necessitates a thorough and comprehensive treatment approach. Early identification and intervention of these difficulties should primarily focus on improving the prelinguistic, oromotor, feeding-related, speech, and language skills of the child. In addition to traditional therapies we should also provide them with recent advancements like oral placement therapy.

SUGGESTED READING

1. Anil MA, Shabnam S, Narayanan S. Feeding and swallowing difficulties in children with Down syndrome. J Intellect Disabil Res. 2019;63(8):992-1014.
2. Bahr D, Rosenfeld-Johnson S. Treatment of children with speech oral placement disorders (OPDs): a paradigm emerges. Commun Disord Quart. 2010;31(3):131-8.
3. Chapman RS, Hesketh LJ. Behavioral phenotype of individuals with Down syndrome. Ment Retard Dev Disabil Res Rev. 2000;6(2):84-95.

4. Finestack L, Abbeduto L. Expressive language profiles of verbally expressive adolescents and young adults with Down syndrome or Fragile X syndrome. J Speech Lang Hear Res. 2010;53:1334-48.
5. Kumin L. Early Communication Skills for Children with Down Syndrome: A Guide for Parents and Professionals. Woodbine House; 2012.
6. Lauteslager P, Vermeer A, Helders P. Disturbances in the motor behaviour of children with Down's syndrome: The need for a theoretical framework. Physiotherapy. 1998;84(1):5-13.
7. Pinter JD, Eliez S, Schmitt JE, Capone GT, Reiss AL. Neuroanatomy of Down's syndrome: A high-resolution MRI study. Am J Psychiatry. 2001;158(10):1659-65.
8. Reed V. An Introduction to Children with Language Disorders. Pearson; 2018.
9. Rupela V, Velleman SL, Andrianopoulos MV. Motor speech skills in children with Down syndrome: A descriptive study. Int J Speech Lang Pathol. 2016;18(5):483-92.
10. Rvachew S, Ohberg A, Savage R. Young children's responses to maximum performance tasks: Preliminary data and recommendations. J Speech Lang Pathol Audiol. 2006;30:6-13.
11. Speech & feeding therapy tools, techniques, & training (ND). TalkTools. https://talktools.com/?srsltid=AfmBOoo MTlT3c JGmpsp2iy_ErDx-k3VqJ2DeyV6Y5BdHYLhLj2 ShtLPD.
12. Shriberg LD, Fourakis M, Hall SD, Karlsson HB, Lohmeier HL, McSweeny JL, et al. Extensions to the Speech Disorders Classification System (SDCS). Clin Linguist Phon. 2010; 24:795-824.

SECTION 4

Definitive Counseling and Inclusion

CHAPTER 22

Counseling: Antenatal to Vocational

Shaji Thomas John, Gayathri K

INTRODUCTION

Counseling should start in the antenatal period itself if there is a suspicion of an abnormality. The predictive value of screening tests should be explained to the patient and confirmatory tests advised if warranted. If the condition is not detected antenatally but is suspected after the child is born, the same should be communicated to the family at birth itself. If the suspicion is not mentioned, the baby may get discharged within a day or two in case of normal delivery and may be reviewed only at 6 weeks, if brought for immunization and follow-up to the same institution.

There have been many instances in our practice in a developing country that the follow-up is done at a local health center, and the karyotype results sent from the place of delivery have not even been collected. Cases have been identified as Down syndrome (DS) even as late as 1 year, only when the child is taken to a pediatrician for some health issue or because of developmental delay. Even cases that have been referred to the DS clinic at birth were brought much later because the parents did not suspect anything wrong with the child, and the benefits of an early intervention were lost. The first 3 years of life is of paramount importance as this is the time that the brain is highly plastic (neuroplasticity of the brain) and interventions made can have the maximum effect.

DIAGNOSIS AND CONFIRMATION

Diagnosis by Gestalt is good enough to initiate the counseling process, but it may be missed or wrongly assumed in the newborn period. Confirmation can be made by fluorescent in situ hybridization (FISH), which takes a shorter time, but karyotyping is essential to find out the type of DS and for proper genetic counseling. All the necessary age-appropriate tests and multidisciplinary consultations should be completed in the shortest possible time and definitive counseling undertaken. Counseling should be done at periodic intervals, as well as when needed during follow-up.

GRIEF AND ACCEPTANCE

We are all aware of the five stages of the "grief model" of Elisabeth Kübler-Ross which states that when coping with an imminent death, or when grieving a loss, or an unanticipated event, individuals will experience denial, anger, bargaining, depression, and acceptance stages. This theory is incomplete and not representative of a number of grief situations including that of DS.

There usually is an intense reaction to having a baby with a disability: Numbness, disappointment, isolation, withdrawal, defensiveness, protest, despair, shock, denial, sadness, anger, self-doubt, humiliation, confusion, disbelief, and guilt. Parents may feel hopeless, a feeling that may be perpetuated by family, friends, or even health professionals.

While this initial grief reaction may become less acute over time, parents of children with DS report re-activation of grief feelings periodically throughout their child's life. This is called "chronic sorrow," an idea proposed in 1962 by Olshansky. And the grief may be reactivated by very minor triggers throughout the child's life, which may be more frequent for mothers than fathers, but both experience chronic sorrow. Damrosch and Perry's study noted that mothers experienced peaks and valleys of crises and adjustment to having a child with DS, whereas fathers experienced more gradual and steady adjustment.

Larson describes an interesting paradox in a study of mothers of children with severe disability. Mothers describe feeling sad and wanting to get rid of the disability from their children even years after the onset of the disability. But at the same time, they also feel content, happy, and loving their child just the way they are. These reactions tell us that the traditional idea of "acceptance" does not apply to parents of children with a disability; instead, their happiness may co-exist with chronic sorrow.

"Meaning-making" theory of bereavement is quite an interesting one in the above context but is highly variable in nature as each person has his own religious beliefs, educational background, cultural influences, family dynamics, intrapersonal characteristics, etc. Two common ways to make meaning out of a loss are *sense-making*, such as fitting the loss into one's spiritual system or changing one's spiritual system in response to the loss, and *silver linings*—seeing the good in a loss.

There are numerous reports of parents describing a silver lining of raising a child with a disability in that it is a growing experience that facilitates a new perspective on life. There are many parents who state that their golden era started after the child with DS was born. Similarly, when mothers of children with DS who were chronically depressed met weekly as a group with a specialist and focused on their grieving, most of them started feeling positive in a year's time, and they recognized that through their experience, they had grown more sensitive to the suffering of others. These mothers were able to derive a meaning from their experience, and this apparently helped them feel better with their situations. Formation of support groups for caretakers also helps in this aspect.

The spiritual and/or existential beliefs of the patient may be explored to gently and indirectly introduce the idea of meaning-making. Some people believe that "Everything happens for a reason" or that "It is the Will of God and He knows best."

COUNSELING AND FOLLOW-UP

As counselors, we tend to be naturally empathetic toward our patients. However, the lives and emotions of our patients are very complex, and thus, we must continually strive to understand and address this complexity, rather than rely solely on our instincts or rigid counseling techniques.

Counseling should be initiated keeping all these in mind. Both parents should be present, ideally along with a support person who is acceptable to the family. This should be done in a counseling room or a room with privacy, and they should be comfortably seated. They should be greeted softly on arrival, establish eye contact, and maintain an open posture. Ample time should be made available to detail the child's status and to answer all the doubts raised. Start the counseling on a positive note, providing accurate information in a balanced manner. Refer to DS as a condition and not as a disease; give importance to the person and not the condition when counseling. The associated conditions should be detailed, and the need for regular follow-up should be stressed. The absence of any disease affecting other systems can be highlighted in a positive manner, especially those systems where a high incidence is noted compared to babies who do not have DS. The possibility of other systemic involvement subsequently (e.g., hypothyroidism) should also be mentioned, and the need for regular checkups should be emphasized. Use an appropriate tone while counseling and be aware of the body language. Allow the attendants to express freely and listen attentively.

The need for early interventional programs should be highlighted. Interventions should be regular and continued till advised. It should be stressed that the mainstay of treatment is the continued therapies as advised, and that there is no medicine that can change the chromosomal status or modify the effect of the chromosomal status as of now. Medicines prescribed for the systemic illnesses, if any, should be continued with regular follow-up. A chart indicating the follow-up to be done at specific ages should preferably be given to the parents so that even if they relocate to another place, they will be aware of when the next follow-up is to be done.

The social issues should be discussed, and their rights should be explained. The basis of management should be a biopsychosocial strategy, together known as healthcare counseling. We should take into account the biological aspect of the high incidence of physical health conditions, the psychological impact on the family and the children themselves, and social aspects such as financial support.

Answers to common questions that are asked should be explained in simple layman's language.

"Why did I have such a baby? Whose fault is it?"

"We are both highly intelligent—how can this happen to us?"

"Is it the fault of our parents or previous life—'Janmam' or 'Janam' for those who believe in re-incarnation?"

"Can my child go to a normal school along with his siblings?"

It is often noted that after you have given a detailed explanation, they ask the same question again and again; partly because their mind goes blank after you start detailing about the condition, and partly because the same doubts keep coming up again and again. This is where the counselor has to be patient, empathetic, understanding, nonjudgmental, and supportive.

Connect them to a DS support group in the locality, which will be of immense help in the months and years to follow. A designated volunteer person from the support group can act as a lay counselor to support the family from the beginning, which will complement the efforts of the doctor.

Recommendations:

- Counseling should be initiated as soon as the diagnosis is suspected as well as after confirmation and full workup. Periodic counseling is required to manage chronic sorrow and to manage issues in between.
- A follow-up chart should be provided to the parents.
- A biopsychosocial strategy should be the basis of management, and the need to continue interventional programs should be stressed.
- Connect them to a local DS support group.

EARLY INTERVENTION/ EDUCATION/VOCATION

Physical therapy with speech stimulation is to be started at birth or at least by 3 months of age. Developmental therapy, occupational therapy, behavior therapy, and cognitive therapy, along with physical therapy and speech therapy, should be initiated at the appropriate time. Psychological evaluation and support should be given as the child grows older. Management of attention deficit hyperactivity disorder (ADHD) and autistic disorders can manifest as early as 2 or 3 years of age, and they should be addressed at the appropriate time. Psychiatric support, especially during adolescent age, is not to be ignored as they can have issues related to sexuality, anxiety, and depression, as in any other adolescent. Support of the family, including siblings, should not be neglected, especially in the initial years of life.

Education in special schools was advocated earlier, but it was found that children with DS who mostly have only mild-to-moderate intellectual disability were not benefited by this, and in fact it deterred their progress, as most of the other children were intellectually more backward compared to these children. Integrated education has been tried where these children are put up in the same classroom as normal children and have to compete with other children for the same educational goals, which may be difficult at times.

Inclusive education is recommended for children with DS, where they go to a normal school but have the support of special teachers and other trained teachers to support them with individualized teaching, where necessary. It is built on the notion that it is more effective for students with special needs to have mixed experience to be more successful in social interactions, leading to further success in life. The philosophy behind the implementation of the inclusion model is that it does not prioritize but still provides for the utilization of special support in the education of students with disabilities.

A special education facility can be started at an early school age, as needed. They can be sent to preschools/ nursery classes or to "Anganvadis." (*Anganvadi is a type of rural child care center in India started by the Indian government in 1975 as part of the Integrated Child Development Services Program. The Hindi word Anganwadi means "courtyard shelter"*)

Children with DS can be enrolled in the first standard of a normal school by 7–8 years of age, based on their intellectual status. Many of the children have pursued vocational courses, and some of them have become graduates. These children are highly trainable and based on their aptitude; vocational training should be started by about 15–17 years (after completion of school). A suitable independent vocation should be encouraged and is preferred to group vocational activities, which should be reserved for children with moderate-to-severe intellectual challenges.

Recommendations:

- Early interventional programs should be started at least by 3 months of age.
- ADHD and autistic behavior should be picked up early and managed.
- Psychiatric support should be given for the adolescents with DS and their parents.
- Inclusive education in a normal school should be advocated.
- Vocational training is to be initiated based on their aptitude.

CONCLUSION

Early diagnosis is essential to plan a proper interventional program. Even a suspicion of the condition may be hinted, so that they are not lost to follow-up due to lack of awareness. A proper counseling should be done as soon as the condition is confirmed. The need for a sustained interventional therapy should be highlighted so that they do not discontinue the therapies after some time. Long-term plans for schooling and vocational training should also be briefly mentioned during the counseling process.

SUGGESTED READING

1. Douglas HA. Promoting meaning—making to help our patients grieve: an exemplar for genetic counselors and other health care professionals. J Genet Couns. 2014;23: 695-700.
2. Ellis JB. Grieving the loss of the perfect child: parents of children with handicaps. Child Adolesc Soc Wo. 1989;6: 259-70.
3. Harvey B. Down's syndrome: a biopsychosocial perspective. Nurs Stand. 2004;18:43-5
4. Holland JM, Neimeyer RA. An examination of stage theory of grief among individuals bereaved by natural and violent causes: a meaning-oriented contribution. Omega. 2010;61:103-20.
5. Kearney PM, Griffin T. Between joy and sorrow: being a parent of a child with developmental disability. J Adv Nurs. 2001;34:582-92.
6. King LA, Scollon CK, Ramsey C, Williams T. Stories of life transition: subjective well-being and ego development in parents of children with down syndrome. J Res Personal. 2000;34:509-36.
7. Kübler-Ross E. On Death and Dying. Routledge; 1973.
8. Larson E. Reframing the meaning of disability to families: the embrace of paradox. Soc Sci Med. 1998;47:865-75.
9. Olshansky S. Chronic sorrow: A response to having a mentally defective child. Soc Casework. 1962;43:190-3.
10. Roche E, Hoey HMCV, Murphy J. Hearing impairment. Medical Management of Children and Adolescents with Down Syndrome in Ireland. 2015:18-20.

CHAPTER 23

Vocational Training and Placement for Persons with Down Syndrome

Jayaraj MK

"A little more patience, a little more love, and a whole lot of understanding: that's the Down Syndrome recipe for a life full of happiness and growth."

INTRODUCTION

There are 200 million people with intellectual disabilities among the total human population. It is not the disability that defines a person, but their capability that does. However, they do need a great deal of attention and support in this regard. All the other sectors of disability are way more privileged, because they are aware of their rights and they unite and fight for their rights. In the case of persons with intellectual challenges, they do not know that they have equal rights. While there are institutions that provide care to those with intellectual disabilities, such support is generally limited till the age of 18. Parents are helpless with no hope. The grown-up individuals with intellectual disabilities are left with their families at that crucial age, in which physical and mental changes are expected to happen in them. Centers which provide support to such individuals to empower them to lead a life with dignity are the need of the hour.

Early detection and intervention are crucial for individuals with intellectual disabilities, regardless of the underlying cause. Early intervention serves as a cornerstone for facilitating the development of essential skills and adaptive behaviors crucial for navigating daily life.

In addition to early intervention, rehabilitation programs play a vital role in supporting the vocational training and placement of intellectually challenged individuals. These programs are designed to equip individuals with the skills, knowledge, and confidence necessary to pursue meaningful employment opportunities. Vocational training focuses on honing specific job-related skills, such as computer literacy, culinary skills, or craftsmanship, tailored to the individual's interests and abilities. Through hands-on training and guidance from experienced professionals, individuals can develop competence and proficiency in their chosen field, enhancing their employability and job prospects. Persons with Down syndrome (DS) are usually only mild to moderately affected, and hence they can be trained to pursue a vocation.

TRANSITION FROM SCHOOL TO WORK

"School to work" transition refers to the critical socio-economic life-changing period between approximately 15 and 24 years of age—a period when young individuals develop and build skills, based on their initial education and training that helps them become productive members of the society.

Transitioning from school to work is a pivotal phase in the lives of young adults, marking a significant shift from structured educational environments to the more dynamic and often unpredictable realm of the workforce. This transition is particularly challenging for persons with DS, who may face difficulties that require careful, tailored approaches to ensure their successful integration into the workplace. Intellectual challenges can vary widely but commonly involve limitations in cognitive functions such as reasoning, problem-solving, and general learning abilities, which are critical in most work settings.

For these individuals, moving into the workforce is not just about finding a job; it is about finding an environment where they can effectively apply their unique skill sets, continue to learn, and grow professionally. Schools typically provide a structured learning environment specifically designed to cater to their educational needs, including specialized support services such as individualized learning plans, therapeutic interventions, and a curriculum adapted to their learning pace and style. However, the workplace often lacks similar accommodations, making the transition potentially stressful and disorienting.

Comprehensive planning for this transition needs to start well before the individual leaves the school system. This planning should involve career counseling, skills assessments, and the development of a transition plan that aligns with the individual's strengths, interests, and the realistic demands of the job market. Additionally, targeted support is crucial and can include job coaching, workplace accommodations, and ongoing vocational training tailored to individual needs. Adaptable strategies are also essential, acknowledging that what works initially may need fine-tuning as the individual and the workplace evolve.

Moreover, this transition is not solely the responsibility of the individual and their family but involves a broader network, including educators, potential employers, and community services, all coordinated to support the individual's journey into the workforce. Such a multifaceted approach ensures that intellectually challenged individuals receive the support they need to overcome barriers, capitalize on their unique talents, and ultimately thrive in a work setting. This is not only beneficial for the individuals themselves but also enriches the workforce with diverse perspectives and capabilities, fostering an inclusive society that values all its members.

ROLE OF VARIOUS STAKEHOLDERS

- *Families:* Families must advocate for their members and provide emotional and practical support as they transition to work environments.
- *Educators:* Teachers and vocational trainers should focus on developing both academic skills and practical vocational skills.
- *Employers:* Employers can create inclusive workplaces by understanding the specific needs and strengths of intellectually challenged employees, adapting training processes, and fostering a supportive work culture.
- *Policy makers:* Governments and local authorities can influence the success of transitions by enacting policies that encourage inclusive hiring practices, subsidize employer accommodations, and fund training programs.

CHALLENGES IN TRANSITIONING FROM SCHOOL TO WORK

- *Educational gaps:* Often, intellectually challenged individuals receive education in specialized settings that are markedly different from typical work environments. This can result in a gap between the skills acquired during school and those required in the workplace.
- *Social and behavioral adaptation:* The social skills and behavioral expectations in a workplace often differ from those taught in school settings. Individuals may struggle with understanding social cues, teamwork, and professional interactions.
- *Limited employment opportunities:* There is often a misconception that intellectually challenged individuals are less capable of performing job tasks. This stigma can lead to fewer employment opportunities and underemployment.
- *Lack of tailored support services:* While schools usually provide structured support, similar support structures in workplaces are rare. The absence of these supports can hinder the ability of these individuals to perform effectively and grow in their roles.

STRATEGIES FOR EFFECTIVE TRANSITION

- *Individualized education programs (IEPs):* Extending the concept of IEPs beyond the school to cover the transition period can provide continuity and support.
- *Collaboration between educational institutions and employers:* Schools, vocational training centers, and potential employers can collaborate to create internship and apprenticeship opportunities.
- *Supportive employment:* This model involves providing job coaches and mentors who help intellectually challenged individuals adapt to the workplace, learn job-specific skills, and navigate challenges.
- *Advocacy and awareness programs:* Raising awareness about the capabilities and needs of intellectually challenged individuals can help reduce stigma and open up more employment opportunities.
- *Use of technology:* Assistive technologies can play a crucial role in helping intellectually challenged individuals perform their job tasks more effectively and independently.

VOCATIONAL TRAINING AND EMPLOYMENT

As individuals with DS reach adulthood, vocational training becomes essential:

- *Job training programs:* These prepare individuals for specific jobs, taking into account their capabilities and interests.

- *Supported employment:* Some individuals may benefit from job coaches or workplace adaptations that allow them to perform their jobs effectively.
- *Entrepreneurial opportunities:* Encouraging and supporting self-employment in areas aligned with their skills and passions.

VOCATIONAL TRAINING AND PLACEMENT OF INDIVIDUALS WITH DOWN SYNDROME

Individuals with DS possess unique talents and abilities that can be nurtured through vocational training programs. Despite facing intellectual challenges, they exhibit a remarkable capacity for learning and contributing to society. Vocational training plays a pivotal role in preparing individuals with DS for employment. These programs focus on developing practical skills, enhancing social interactions, and fostering independence. By tailoring training to their unique needs and abilities, individuals with DS can acquire the necessary competencies to succeed in various job roles.

Vocational training for individuals with DS helps to develop a diverse range of skills including communication, problem-solving, and technical abilities. It also trains them to be independent and become more self-sufficient, enhancing their overall quality of life. In addition, it helps them in social integration, and employment provides individuals with DS a sense of purpose and belonging.

CHALLENGES AND BARRIERS

Despite the numerous benefits of vocational training, individuals with DS often encounter challenges and barriers in securing employment. Some of the key challenges include:

- *Stigma and discrimination:* Negative stereotypes and misconceptions about individuals with DS can lead to discrimination in the workplace.
- *Limited opportunities:* Limited availability of job placements tailored to the abilities of individuals with DS can hinder their access to meaningful employment opportunities.
- *Support needs:* They may require additional support and accommodations in the workplace to succeed, without which they may struggle to navigate job responsibilities and social interactions.
- *Transition planning:* Effective transition planning is essential for these individuals as they move from school to adulthood.

STRATEGIES FOR SUCCESSFUL PLACEMENT OF INDIVIDUALS WITH DOWN SYNDROME

Education and Advocacy

Educational campaigns should focus on both the public and specific stakeholders such as business leaders, HR professionals, and educators. These efforts aim to illuminate the unique strengths and contributions that individuals with DS can bring to the workforce, debunk myths and misconceptions, and highlight success stories.

Awareness workshops, seminars, and media campaigns can be organized to educate potential employers about the capabilities of individuals with DS, focusing on their potential rather than their limitations. Offering inclusion training for current employees about diversity and inclusion can foster a more welcoming environment.

Tailored Support Services

To facilitate successful employment outcomes, providing individualized support services is essential. These services need to be adaptable to meet the specific requirements of each individual with DS. It includes job coaching and implementing technology solutions that assist them in performing their job tasks. Adjustments such as flexible work schedules, modified job responsibilities, or physical workspace modifications are necessary to support the unique needs of these employees.

Collaboration with Employers

Building strong partnerships with employers is fundamental to securing meaningful employment opportunities for individuals with DS. Hiring individuals with DS can be part of the corporate social responsibility of companies, as these initiatives demonstrate a commitment to social values and diversity. Establishing a feedback loop with employers allows for continuous improvement in support services and accommodations.

Transition Planning

Effective transition planning from educational settings to the workplace is vital for individuals with DS. This process should start early and involve a coordinated effort among educators, vocational counselors, families, and potential employers.

NATURE OF JOBS FOR INDIVIDUALS WITH DOWN SYNDROME

In recent years, societal views on DS have shifted significantly. From once limiting expectations to now embracing the potential of every individual, the workplace has become a new frontier for inclusivity and empowerment. Historically, individuals with DS were often excluded from the workforce, based on misconceptions about their abilities. However, as understanding and support have improved, so have the employment opportunities. Education and vocational training tailored to individuals with DS have become more prevalent, providing the skills needed to enter various job roles.

SECTORS EMBRACING INCLUSIVITY

- *Retail and hospitality:* These sectors are particularly suited to individuals with DS, as they often involve repetitive tasks and interaction with customers, where individuals can excel with their often-noted friendly and approachable demeanor.
- *Corporate settings:* There is a growing trend of including people with DS in corporate environments. This includes roles in administrative support, document scanning, and data entry.
- *Creative arts:* The arts provide a flexible and expressive outlet for individuals with DS. From acting and dancing to participating in art and music therapy sessions, these fields allow them to express themselves and engage with the community.
- *Agriculture and gardening:* Jobs in these fields offer great environments for individuals who may prefer less crowded, quiet spaces. Tasks such as planting, caring for animals, and maintaining spaces can be highly rewarding and well-suited to their abilities.
- *Tech and innovation:* Some organizations are pioneering roles in technology for individuals with DS. Through especially designed training programs, they are able to take on roles in software testing, where attention to detail is crucial.

TYPES OF EMPLOYMENT OPTIONS FOR INDIVIDUALS WITH DOWN SYNDROME

In general, there are three types of employment options available to individuals with DS: Competitive, supported, and sheltered.

Competitive Employment

Competitive employment refers to jobs that are available in the general labor market, where these individuals compete with others (with or without disabilities) for the same positions based on their skills and qualifications. These positions are usually not modified specifically for persons with disabilities and offer the same wages and benefits as those offered to other employees performing similar roles.

The challenges for such employment include finding employers willing to hire individuals with DS, navigating competitive interview and selection processes, as well as requiring certain levels of independence and job-specific skills.

The benefits are enhanced self-esteem with a sense of accomplishment, better social integration and interpersonal skills, and financial independence.

Supported Employment

Supported employment is designed to help individuals with disabilities, including DS, who need substantial support to succeed in a work environment. This type of employment includes job coaches, workplace adjustments, and ongoing support tailored to the individual's needs.

The challenges are dependence on support services for success and limited availability of job coaches or resources in some regions.

The benefits are that it facilitates employment in a wider range of job settings, provides a structured environment that can maximize the individual's job performance, and helps build confidence and skills in a supportive setting.

Sheltered Employment

Sheltered employment typically takes place in workshops or specialized facilities where only individuals with disabilities are employed. These settings provide highly structured environments where individuals can work on simple assembly tasks, packaging, or other types of work designed to accommodate their abilities.

The challenges include limited interaction with the broader community and lower wages compared to competitive or even some supported employment settings. They can be seen as segregative rather than integrative.

The benefits are that they provide a safe and controlled work environment, allow individuals who may not thrive in competitive or supported employment to work and earn an income, and help develop work habits and skills that could potentially be transferable to other employment settings.

POSSIBLE WAYS TO ADDRESS THE ISSUES OF INTELLECTUALLY CHALLENGED INDIVIDUALS IN DEVELOPING COUNTRIES

In developing countries, intellectually challenged individuals encounter a myriad of obstacles when seeking the support and services essential for their well-being. The present scenario is characterized by persistent barriers to integration, education, and employment, exacerbated by limited resources, a shortage of trained professionals, and societal stigma. Addressing these challenges requires concerted efforts to enhance access to education, create inclusive employment opportunities, and expand support services for intellectually challenged individuals and their families. Many individuals with DS are independently employed all over the country and leading a gratifying life of happiness and growth, with minimal external support.

PLACEMENT PROCEDURE THAT CAN BE ADOPTED FROM THE SUCCESSFUL MODEL OF URALUNGAL LABOUR CONTRACT CO-OPERATIVE SOCIETY FOUNDATION IN KERALA

Adequate training and guidance can enhance their skill and thereby help them to earn a livelihood. Studies show that 80% of individuals with intellectual challenges are employable if they are provided with proper training. After completing their primary education up to the age of 18, vocational training is a must for individuals with disabilities. Therefore, it is imperative to provide employment opportunities to the differently-abled individuals.

- *Assessment and evaluation:* The placement process begins with a thorough assessment conducted by specialized educators. Through interviews, observations, and standardized assessments, a comprehensive profile of each trainee is meticulously crafted. This assessment is not only for the individuals with intellectual challenges but also involves their families. With a profound understanding of each trainee's unique attributes, challenges, and goals, we can tailor training and support programs with precision.
- *Selection and in-house vocational training:* Based on the assessment results, individuals with intellectual challenges are selected, and they undergo in-house vocational training at UL Care Nayanar Sadanam. The training aims to enhance their skills and prepare them for future employment opportunities.
- *On-the-job training placement:* After completing in-house vocational training, individuals are placed in various public and private sector institutions for on-the-job training. This phase is crucial as it provides real-world work experience and allows them to apply the skills they have learned. They are paid monthly salary for their duties. The goal is to facilitate their integration into the workforce and promote self-sufficiency.
- *Regular monitoring and follow-ups:* The support does not end with job placement. Special educators from UL Care Nayanar Sadanam continue to play an active role by conducting regular monitoring and follow-up visits to the placement institutions. This ongoing support ensures that the individuals are adapting well to their work environment and receiving the necessary assistance.
- *Feedback collection from employers:* Feedback is a vital component of the placement process. This feedback helps assess the individual's performance and identify areas for improvement. It also helps strengthen the collaboration between the institution and the employer organizations.

IN-HOUSE JOB TRAINING

Recognizing that not all individuals at UL Care Nayanar Sadanam may be ready or able to work outside the institution, Uralungal Labour Contract Co-operative Society (ULCCS) Foundation takes a holistic approach. It offers in-house jobs, where individuals with intellectual challenges engage in creative activities such as making bead necklaces, bags, and small crafts, under the guidance of special educators. This approach taps into their creativity, providing a sense of purpose and accomplishment. The products created by them are made available for sale at "Sargasheshi" Handicrafts Shop, an initiative by the ULCCS Foundation and the Down Syndrome Trust (DoST) that focuses on empowering women with DS.

"Sargasheshi" a Venture for Women with Down Syndrome

People with intellectual disability are a vulnerable group not properly addressed by the society. Much worse is the case of women with intellectual disability. Additional considerations about their gender-specific needs and vulnerabilities must be considered.

"Sargasheshi" is a handicrafts showroom in Kozhikode District of Kerala run by women with DS. There are exquisite crafts that make the shop beautiful. But what makes it more beautiful are the women who run the shop. The prime objective of the project is to provide a livelihood for women with DS. A supervisor, who is also an experienced special educator, helps them out there and also deals with the accounts.

"Sargasheshi" challenges the stereotypes by demonstrating that individuals with DS are capable of contributing meaningfully to society. Through training and support, the women involved in the project develop valuable skills in handicraft production, fostering a sense of independence and self-worth. As the first of its kind in India, "Sargasheshi" serves as a model for future initiatives seeking to empower marginalized communities and promote social change through creativity and collaboration.

CONCLUSION

In the pursuit of inclusivity and empowerment, vocational training and placement programs serve as invaluable pathways for individuals with DS, offering them opportunities to develop skills, independence, and a sense of purpose. These programs not only equip individuals with practical abilities but also foster dignity and belonging within society. However, the journey toward inclusive empowerment extends beyond vocational training—it requires concerted efforts to address systemic barriers and cultivate a culture of acceptance and support. While significant strides have been made globally to support individuals with DS, the challenges faced by intellectually challenged individuals in developing countries persist. Central to the success of this mission is a commitment to dignity, inclusion, and empowerment for all individuals. Through the initiation of a dedicated mission activity inspired by global models and grounded in cooperative principles, one should create a society where all individuals, regardless of ability, can thrive and contribute meaningfully to their communities.

SUGGESTED READING

1. Billet S, Fenwick T, Somerville M. (Eds). "Work, Subjectivity, and Learning: Understanding Learning Through Working Life". Springer 2006.
2. Jayaraj MK. "Pertaining to the issues of persons with intellectual disabilities". MK Jayaraj Commission Report 2016.
3. Lauglo J, Maclean R (Eds). "Vocationalisation of Secondary Education Revisited". Springer 2005.
4. Pruthvish S. "Vocational Training and Employment of Persons with Disability, New Delhi". National Institute of Public Cooperation and Child Development, 2006.
5. Rusch FR, Hughes C. "Supported Employment: Models, Methods, and Issues." Baltimore: Paul H Brookes Publishing Co., 2006.
6. Sengupta AK. "Vocational Rehabilitation of Disabled in India: Principles and Practice, Bangalore. Niruta Publications, 2017.
7. Test DW. "Evidence Based Instructional Strategies for Transition". Baltimore, MD: Paul H Brookes Publishing Co., 2012.
8. Wehman P, Inge KJ, Revell WG, Brooke VA. "Real Work for Real Pay: Inclusive Employment for People with Disabilities." Baltimore, MD: Paul H Brookes Publishing Co., 2007.
9. Wehman P, Kregel J. "Functional Curriculum for Elementary, Middle, and Secondary Age Students with Special Needs". (3rd Edn.) Austin, TX: PRO-ED, 2012.

CHAPTER 24

Community-based Rehabilitation for Neurodevelopmental Disorders

Krishnakumar P

INTRODUCTION

The term rehabilitation refers to restoring skills lost due to illnesses or injuries. In children with neurodevelopmental disorders (NDDs), interventions generally focus on helping the child to attain skills that are not attained or delayed or rarely skills that have been lost over time. Hence, it is argued that the term habilitation is better suited to interventions for children with NDD and not rehabilitation. The World Health Organization (WHO) defines rehabilitation as "a set of interventions to optimize functioning and reduce disability in individuals with health conditions in their interaction with the living environment." Hence, it is not inappropriate to use the term rehabilitation in connection with interventions for NDDs in children and the term is used in this paper in this sense.

There was a time when people with serious mental illnesses and disabilities were segregated and ostracized as "possessed with demons or evil spirits." The attitude of society toward disability changed gradually with better understanding of the functioning of the human body and increasing concerns about human rights. During the last half of the 19th century and the first half of the 20th century, the focus shifted to institutional care of individuals with neurodisabilities, and institutions to care for people with chronic mental illnesses and neurodisabilities flourished. Rehabilitation services for disabilities were also centered on an institutional approach and most often the services were available in city-based institutions.

COMMUNITY-BASED REHABILITATION

There was a paradigm shift in the attitude toward neurodisability during the latter part of the 20th century, with focus on community-based care and community-based rehabilitation (CBR) services. In many parts of the world, especially in low- and middle-income countries like India, rehabilitation services are still limited largely to city-based institutions and, that too grossly inadequate. Optimum rehabilitation services are often hampered by lack of qualified rehabilitation professionals and other resources. Affordability, lack of awareness, stigma, and accessibility issues compel many parents to discontinue remedial therapy, resulting in persistent disabilities.

In 1976, the WHO introduced the concept of CBR as the effective strategy to provide rehabilitation services to people with disabilities in low- and middle-income countries. The WHO defines CBR as a "strategy within general community development for the rehabilitation, equalization of opportunities, poverty reduction, and social inclusion of people with disabilities". In the broader sense, CBR is intended for both persons with disabilities (PWDs), their families, and caregivers. The services are to be delivered at the local community level as a part of the local community development initiatives. Ideally, CBR activities are implemented with active involvement of PWDs, their families, and caretakers with support from nongovernment organizations (NGOs) or government agencies and should address issues related to health, education, livelihood, social inclusion, and empowerment either alone or together. Effectiveness and success of CBR depends on need based and targeted planning to address locally relevant issues.

The WHO had introduced the concept of task shifting or task sharing to overcome the shortage of health professionals and reduce the treatment gap in neuropsychological disorders. Task shifting or task sharing is a strategy, where less skilled health workers are trained to provide specialized services and perform specialized tasks that are normally carried out by specialists. CBR guidelines are formulated adopting the principles of task shifting for the effective utilization of available resources **(Box 1)**.

Community-based rehabilitation is not just disability reduction and providing medical aid or assistive devices, but it is a strategy to attain community-based inclusive

BOX. 1: Components of a community-based rehabilitation program (WHO, 2010).

- *Health:*
  - Promotion
  - Prevention
  - Medical care
  - Rehabilitation
  - Assistive devices
- *Education:*
  - Early childhood
  - Primary
  - Secondary and higher
  - Nonformal education
  - Lifelong learning
- *Livelihood:*
  - Skill development
  - Self-employment
  - Wage employment
  - Financial services
  - Social protection
- *Social inclusion:*
  - Personal assistance
  - Relationship, marriage, and family
  - Culture and arts
  - Recreation, leisure, and sports
  - Justice
- *Empowerment:*
  - Advocacy and communication
  - Community mobilization
  - Political participation
  - Self-help groups
  - Disabled people's organizations

development (CBID) for people with disabilities. It was argued that the term CBR stresses on the medical aspects of rehabilitation and hence is reductionistic. CBID is a rights-based approach for inclusive development of people with disabilities and CBR should be planned with this concept in mind.

Health-related activities form one of the core components of the CBR programs and should include health promotion, timely medical care, rehabilitation activities, and assistive devices. Educational planning for children with disabilities should address issues related to early childhood education as well as primary, secondary, and higher education. Provision for nonformal education and lifelong learning should be incorporated in CBR. CBR should help the persons with disabilities become self-reliant and to provide for their own livelihood. Skill development, self-employment programs, financial services, and social protection activities should be planned accordingly. The social dimension of CBR includes personal assistance, relationship, marriage, family, culture and arts, recreation, sports, leisure, and justice. CBR should facilitate formation of self-help groups and disabled people's organizations for better community mobilization and political participation.

COMMUNITY-BASED REHABILITATION IN THE INDIAN CONTEXT: OUR EXPERIENCE

Planning CBR for different types of NDD on an individual basis is not feasible and, not recommended since it may lead to further segregation. The specific needs of children with different types of disorders and varying degrees of disabilities should be addressed while planning CBR. Specific activities or programs for children with Down syndrome could be incorporated in the general programs for NDD.

Community-based rehabilitation for children with developmental problems should include components of early detection, early intervention, preschool education, school education, and vocational training. In the present context, children with DS fail to get regular remedial therapy due to accessibility and affordability issues. Early identification and regular remedial therapy, often for prolonged periods, involving a multidisciplinary team of rehabilitation professionals, are essential for optimum improvement.

Lack of trained manpower is one of the major hurdles in implementing a comprehensive rehabilitation program for children with NDDs in low- and middle-income countries, apart from financial constraints. Studies have shown that trained lay health workers could provide early detection and intervention services for NDDs in resource poor settings adhering to the principles of task sharing or task shifting. In our experience, Anganwadi* teachers, who attended a short-term structured training program were able to identify children under 3 years with developmental delay and to provide follow-up intervention in the local Anganwadi, to supplement institution-based professional intervention. Digital technologies like mobile App were found to help both parents and health workers to identify

**Anganwadi is a government-sponsored child-care and mother-care development programmes in India at the village level started in 1975 as part of the Integrated Child Development Services program to combat child hunger and malnutrition. It caters to children in the 0–6 age group.*

children with developmental delays as early as 6 months. In another experimental project we found that regular institution-based remedial therapy by rehabilitation professionals for 3 days a week followed by Anganwadi-based intervention for the next 3 days is more effective than conventional remedial therapy.

Accessibility to city-based centers that provide remedial therapy services is another major issue for children coming from remote villages and many drop out from regular therapy sessions resulting in poor outcome. We have found that a mobile developmental disability team could be able to address this issue to a certain extent. The mobile intervention team, comprising clinical psychologist, speech therapist, developmental therapist, and special educator visited prefixed days on selected government-owned community health centers or centers supported by local NGOs and provided early detection and early intervention services. As part of the project, local Anganwadi teachers were given training to identify and refer children with developmental delay. After detailed evaluation and treatment plan from the apex center, children availed remedial therapy services from the mobile units along with Anganwadi-based intervention. It was found that Anganwadi-based intervention could be made more effective by providing the services of a special educator in addition to the regular staff.

Inclusive education with no segregation and need-based individualized curriculum is recommended for school education of children with NDD, especially DS. Implementation of inclusive education is met with many hurdles, especially in low- and middle-income countries, like lack of infrastructure and manpower. Children with DS, especially with moderate to severe intellectual disability, often do not get the necessary care and support in the regular classroom and special schools or special needs school continues to be mainstay of education of children with special needs in our country. We found that utilizing one or more classrooms in a regular school to provide training to children with NDD facilitated mutual interaction between students and helped to reduce stigma and segregation. Regular school students also benefited since the interaction with children with special needs helped to develop empathy and understanding. An arrangement where the special needs schools are linked to regular schools to function as collaborative institutions with adequate opportunity for mutual interaction will be a practical solution for the problem of school education of children with intellectual disability.

It is suggested that the government should initiate vertical ("top to bottom") programs to address the rehabilitation needs of persons with disabilities if no active intervention programs are available in the community. Even though the above programs were government funded top to bottom programs organized with aim to fill in the gaps in the rehabilitation services for children with NDD including DS, as the programs evolved many components of CBR could be incorporated. Training and empowerment activities for parents, health workers, and community volunteers organized as part of the programs helped to promote advocacy and human rights perspective of disability and in many places the local NGOs were motivated to take up CBR activities.

CONCLUSION

Community-based rehabilitation is a community-driven approach which focuses on improving access to health, education, livelihood, social inclusion, and empowerment. CBR involves families, local health workers, educators, and community members in providing care and support. It promotes early identification, therapy, inclusive education, and vocational training tailored to each individual's needs. The approach helps reduce stigma and encourages participation in everyday community life. By using local resources and building awareness, CBR offers a sustainable and inclusive solution for managing NDDs.

SUGGESTED READING

1. Butura AM, Ryan GK, Shakespeare T, Ogunmola O, Omobowale O, Greenley R, et al. Community-based rehabilitation for people with psychosocial disabilities in low- and middle-income countries: a systematic review of the grey literature. Int J Ment Health Syst. 2024; 18(1):13.
2. De Groote W. Concept changes and standardizing tools in community-based rehabilitation. Phys Med Rehabil Clin N Am. 2019;30:709-21.
3. Divan G, Vajaratkar V, Cardozo P, Huzurbazar S, Verma M, Howarth E, et al. The feasibility and effectiveness of pass plus, A lay health worker delivered comprehensive intervention for autism spectrum disorders: Pilot RCT in a rural low and middle income country setting. Autism Res. 2019;12:328-39
4. Iemmi V, Kumar KS, Blanchet K, Gibson L, Hartley S, Murthy GVS, et al. Community-based rehabilitation for

people with physical and mental disabilities in low- and middle-income countries. Cochrane Database Syst Rev. 2017;2017(3):CD010617.
5. Nair MK, Princly P, Leena ML, Swapna S, Kumari I L, Preethi R, et al. CDC Kerala 17: Early detection of developmental delay/disability among children below 3 y in Kerala—a cross-sectional survey. Indian J Pediatr. 2014;81(Suppl 2):S156-60.
6. World Health Organization. CBR: a strategy for rehabilitation, equalization of opportunities, poverty reduction and social inclusion of people with disabilities. Geneva: World Health Organization; 2004.
7. World Health Organization. Community-based rehabilitation: CBR guidelines—introductory booklet. Geneva: World Health Organization; 2010. p. 7.
8. WHO, mhGAP. mhGAP Intervention Guide for Mental, Neurological and Substance Use Disorders in Non-specialized Health Settings. Geneva, Switzerland: WHO; 2010.

SECTION

5 Legal Aspects and the Future

CHAPTER 25

Controversies in Management of Down Syndrome

Shaji Thomas John

INTRODUCTION

Controversial therapies have been tried in many chronic diseases and developmental disabilities. It may be because there are no standard treatment guidelines, or because of the chronicity of the problem, or the societal pressures on the families to try various modes of therapies. Various therapies have been tried in the past all over the world but many of them lack sufficient scientific evidence or raise ethical issues.

DRUGS/SUPPLEMENTS/THERAPIES

Nutritional supplements and vitamin therapy: Megavitamin therapy using high doses of vitamins, particularly vitamin B_6, vitamin A, C, E, and folic acid, to improve cognitive function in individuals with Down syndrome (DS) has been tried. A variety of commercial supplements, often marketed as "nutraceuticals" or "nutritional therapies", claimed to enhance cognitive abilities or overall health. These supplements include high dose of antioxidants (omega-3 fatty acid), amino acids, docosahexaenoic acid (DHA), dimethyl sulfoxide (DMSO), trace elements such as selenium, zinc, manganese, copper, and other substances. They are based on the belief that a higher amount of these supplemental agents is required for the body to maintain the normal metabolic processes in these individuals. The efficacy and safety of these supplements are not well-established, and excessive intake of certain vitamins can be harmful. They are also not regulated by health authorities, raising concerns about their use. However, normal supplement of vitamins and trace elements may be beneficial in children with DS.

Nootropics: Piracetam is a nootropic (cognitive enhancer) that has been used for the treatment of cognitive impairments. Some studies have explored its use in individuals with DS, but the results have been inconclusive, and the drug is not approved for this purpose. Other cognitive enhancers have also been explored as potential treatments for DS, but their use remains controversial due to limited evidence and potential risks.

Other drugs: Green tea extracts containing epigallocatechin-3-gallate (EGCG), other antioxidants, and fluoxetine are being tried in mice models and reported to be promising. Donepezil had been advocated in young adults with DS as per some studies to prevent the occurrence of Alzheimer disease. It has been reported to improve the mental status of active children who became dull in their 30s. But all these do not have sufficient scientific backing.

Stem cell therapy: The use of stem cells to treat DS is highly controversial and remains largely experimental. Some clinics offer stem cell treatments with the claim that they can improve cognitive function or physical health in individuals with DS. However, there is no credible scientific evidence to support these claims, and such treatments may pose significant risks, including the potential for tumor formation and other complications. The use of stem cells, especially when derived from embryos, also raises ethical issues. Additionally, the promotion of unproven stem cell therapies can exploit the hopes and fears of families, leading to significant financial and emotional costs without guaranteed benefits.

Biomedical therapies: The use of hormone therapies, such as growth hormone or thyroid hormone supplementation, to treat DS have been tried. Thyroid hormone was used as a brain stimulant in small doses in euthyroid individuals and growth hormone to improve the height and general wellbeing. While thyroid hormone replacement is standard for individuals with hypothyroidism, the use of growth hormone and other hormones without clear medical indications is controversial and may carry risks.

Chelation therapy, which is typically used to remove heavy metals from the body, has been controversially suggested for treating DS under the theory that it might "detoxify" the body and improve cognitive function. This theory is not supported by scientific evidence, and chelation therapy can be dangerous, leading to serious side effects such as kidney damage and even death.

Hyperbaric oxygen therapy (HBOT): HBOT involves breathing pure oxygen in a pressurized chamber and has been proposed as a treatment for cognitive deficits in DS. However, the scientific evidence supporting its effectiveness is weak, and the treatment is expensive and potentially risky.

Behavioral and cognitive training programs: Some controversial training programs claim to significantly enhance cognitive abilities in individuals with DS through specialized training regimens. While early intervention and education are crucial, certain programs may make exaggerated claims that are not backed by scientific research, potentially leading to false hope and unnecessary financial burdens for families.

ALTERNATIVE AND COMPLEMENTARY MEDICINE

Various herbal and homeopathic remedies have been marketed as treatments for DS. These treatments often lack scientific validation and can pose risks due to unknown interactions with other medications or underlying health conditions. Approaches such as energy healing, orthomolecular therapy, acupuncture, and other alternative therapies have been suggested by some as treatments for DS. While these therapies may offer some benefits in terms of relaxation or stress reduction, they are not supported by scientific evidence as effective treatments for the cognitive or developmental aspects of DS.

While many of these treatments have been proposed with the intention of improving the lives of individuals with DS, they often lack solid scientific backing and can pose significant risks. It is essential for families and caregivers to rely on evidence-based interventions and to consult with medical professionals before pursuing any treatment. The focus should remain on supportive care, early intervention, and therapies that are proven to enhance the quality of life for individuals with DS.

CONTROVERSIAL SURGICAL PROCEDURES

Plastic surgery to normalize the major physical stigmata of DS has been performed most frequently in Europe. There are major philosophical issues involved, and there is, as yet, not enough information to allow the development of a cost-benefit analysis.

Tubal ligation for women with DS had been debated since they are more prone for abuse and unplanned pregnancies with issues related to offsprings of women with DS. So also, hysterectomy used to be advocated by some not only to prevent conception but also for the management of monthly periods. It was assumed that such people were not able to take care of themselves or their children, nor able to educate them, and should not be allowed to risk transmitting their intellectual disability to offspring. But these children can be well trained to handle the monthly periods, and the above procedures in an intellectually subnormal person who is not capable of giving a proper consent are not justifiable and raise many ethical issues. Moreover, these procedures do not prevent sexually transmitted diseases (STDs), and it is better to teach them about prevention of STDs and birth control where applicable.

TERMINATION OF A PREGNANCY WHEN DIAGNOSED

The choice to continue or terminate a pregnancy after a diagnosis of DS is an individual decision. There is no universally "right" answer, as the decision ultimately depends on the values, beliefs, and circumstances of the individual or couple involved. It is essential that the decision is made based on a thorough understanding of the condition, consideration of personal and family values, and after seeking appropriate medical advice and counseling. Respect for the autonomy of the individuals involved is paramount, and they should be supported regardless of the choice they make.

Factors to be considered: The nature of the condition should be understood—the health issues involved and challenges ahead. Many people with DS lead fulfilling lives, and advancements in medical care, education, and social inclusion have significantly improved their life expectancy and quality of life. Most individuals with DS attend school, and some hold jobs, and maintain meaningful relationships.

Personal beliefs and values should be taken into consideration. Some people may have strong ethical or religious beliefs that influence their decision regarding termination. For some, the idea of terminating a pregnancy due to a genetic condition may conflict with their beliefs about the sanctity of life. The values and priorities of the family, including how they view disability and the role they see for themselves in raising a child with special needs, are crucial factors in the decision-making process. Deciding whether to continue or terminate a pregnancy can be emotionally challenging. It is important to consider the emotional impact on the parents and family, both in the short-term and long-term aspects. Access to a strong support network, including family, friends, and healthcare professionals, can play a significant role in the decision-making process and in managing the potential challenges of raising a child with DS.

Raising a child with DS may require additional resources, including specialized medical care, educational support, and potentially lifelong care. The availability of these resources, as well as the family's financial and social support systems, can influence the decision. Parents may consider the long-term care needs of a child with DS, including the status as the parents age and caregiving responsibilities in the future.

Legal consideration: The legal framework surrounding abortion varies from country to country. It may be permitted only within certain gestational limits. In some places, access to abortion may be more restricted. Some people argue that if termination be legalized for conditions like DS, then later on termination could be demanded for even minor abnormalities detected antenatally.

The ultimate decision rests with the parents within the legal framework of the country.

CONCLUSION

Various controversial therapies have been tried all over the world due to the lack of standard treatment guidelines in the past. Some of them may be of benefit in selected cases, but most of them do not have any scientific backing. When in doubt, it is always best for the family to discuss the pros and cons with the treating physician and make an informed decision. This should take into account financial considerations, available social support systems, religious values, family priorities, and must be made within the legal framework of the country.

SUGGESTED READING

1. Gerald S. Golden; Controversies in Therapies for Children with Down Syndrome. Pediatr Rev October. 1984;6(4): 116-20.
2. Monteiro S, Soares S, Matos IS, Machado L, Mendes DG, Coutinho AC. Promising therapeutic approaches in Down Syndrome: addressing parents' doubts. Pediatr Oncall. 2024;21(1).

CHAPTER 26

Legal Aspects and Decision Making

Shaji Thomas John

INTRODUCTION

Management of Down syndrome (DS) had always been intertwined with controversies. The life span of a child with DS was considered to be <10 years in the early 20th century and even as late as in 1980 it was considered to be <25 years. Hence, active management, especially medical treatment in a child who was intellectually subnormal was not advocated; as it was considered a waste on the national exchequer and only served to prolong the hardships of the caretakers.

On April 9th 1982, in Bloomington in the state of Indiana in USA, a baby with DS was born who also had esophageal atresia. The baby was advised operation for correction of esophageal atresia but there was objection from some members of the medical fraternity because the child had DS and would be "mentally retarded". The matter was taken up for presentation to the US Supreme Court Justice John Paul Stevens. But before the case could be heard, the baby died on 15th April at 6 days of age as a result of dehydration and pneumonia. The baby had been named Baby Doe and this incident brought in the "Baby Doe Law" or the "Baby Doe Amendment" to the Child Abuse Law in the US. Later the "Baby Doe Rules" came in as part of the 1988 "Revision of the Child Abuse Prevention and Treatment Act" (CAPTA).

In 1995, a 34-year-old woman "SJ" with DS and congenital heart disease who later developed heart failure was recommended heart transplantation. But she was denied the procedure despite being approved by the California Medicaid. She underwent a successful transplantation only after a successful lawsuit. Historically, organ transplantation in DS was considered a contraindication till the above landmark case.

In yet another noteworthy case, Baby B, a newborn with DS had intestinal obstruction which would have been fatal unless treated. Her parents refused to consent to the operation, as it was believed that even if the operation was carried out, her life expectancy would be only 20–30 years. They decided that it would be in the interests of the child to allow her to die rather than to live physically and mentally handicapped. But the doctor contacted the local authority who made the baby a ward of court and got the court to authorize the operation. The attending surgeon who respected the wishes of the parents declined to carry it out. And the local authority went back to the court.

The verdict of the court was as noted below:

> *"... while great weight ought to be given to the views of the parents they are not the views which must necessarily prevail. ... Fortunately or unfortunately, in this particular case the decision no longer lies with the parents or with the doctors, but lies with the court. ... the duty of the court is to decide whether it is in the interests of the child ... (which is to decide) whether the life of this child is demonstrably going to be so awful that in effect the child must be condemned to die, or whether the life of this child is still so imponderable that it would be wrong for her to be condemned to die. There may be cases ... where the life of the child is so bound to be full of pain and suffering that the court might be driven to a different conclusion, but in the present case the choice which lies before the court is this: whether to allow an operation to take place which may result in the child living for 20 or 30 years as a Mongoloid, or whether to terminate the life of a Mongoloid child because she also has an intestinal complaint. Faced with that choice I have no doubt that it is the duty of this court to decide that the child must live".*

PERSONS WITH DISABILITIES (EQUAL OPPORTUNITIES, PROTECTION OF RIGHTS, AND FULL PARTICIPATION) ACT, 1995

The "Persons with Disabilities (Equal Opportunities, Protection of Rights, and Full Participation) Act, 1995" by the Government of India, came into enforcement on February 7, 1996. This law was brought in to ensure equal opportunities for people with disabilities and their full participation in the nation building. The Act provides for both preventive and promotional aspects of rehabilitation like education, employment and vocational training, reservation, research and manpower development, creation of barrier-free environment, rehabilitation of persons with disability, unemployment and establishment of homes for persons with severe disability, etc. This Act has been replaced by the RPwD Act, 2016.

THE NATIONAL TRUST ACT, 1999

The National Trust Act, 1999 was passed for the welfare of persons with autism, cerebral palsy, mental retardation, and multiple disabilities by the Ministry of Social Justice and Empowerment, Government of India. Clause 10(a) of the Act mentions: To enable and empower persons with disabilities to live as independently and as fully as possible within and as close to the community to which they belong.

Later the *National Trust Rules* came in 2000 and the *National Trust Regulations* in 2001. The regulations ensure that individuals with these disabilities receive the support they need through a well-structured system of care, guardianship, and welfare programs, promoting their inclusion and participation in society. The provision for establishing a legal guardianship to provide a legal framework for the appointment of guardians for persons with disabilities who require assistance in managing their personal affairs was highlighted. The regulations also provide for legal assistance to persons with disabilities in cases where their rights are being violated.

Various welfare schemes like *Samarth Scheme* to provide residential facilities (Samarth Centers) for persons with disabilities who do not have family support, *Niramaya Scheme* to provide health insurance coverage for persons with disabilities and *Sahyogi Scheme* to give training for caregivers of persons with disabilities were the noteworthy ones in addition to various other schemes.

THE UNITED NATIONS CONVENTION ON THE RIGHTS OF PERSONS WITH DISABILITIES

The *United Nations Convention on the Rights of Persons with Disabilities (UNCRPD)* came in 2006 to promote, protect, and ensure the full and equal enjoyment of all human rights and fundamental freedoms by all persons with disabilities, and to promote respect for their inherent dignity. (Article 1) Some of the features stressed are as follows:

Article 6: Ensure the equal rights and advancement of women and girls with disabilities.

Article 7: Protect children with disabilities.

Article 10: Countries are to guarantee that persons with disabilities enjoy their inherent right to life on an equal basis with others (as of March 2025 there are 164 countries as signatories to the Convention; and 182 countries have ratified it)

Article 25: Provide persons with disabilities with the same range, quality, and standard of free or affordable health care and programs as provided to other persons. Prevent discriminatory denial of health care or health services or food and fluids on the basis of disability. Persons with disabilities have the right to the highest attainable standard of health without discrimination on the basis of disability.

A country that ratifies the convention on the Rights of Persons with Disabilities (RPwD) agrees to be legally bound to treat persons with disabilities as subjects of the law with clearly defined rights as any other person. Ratifying countries will have to adapt their domestic legislation to the international standards laid out in the treaty.

RIGHTS OF PERSONS WITH DISABILITIES ACT, 2016

The *Rights of Persons with Disabilities Act, 2016 (RPwD Act, 2016)* is a comprehensive law in India that aims to protect the rights and promote the inclusion of persons with disabilities (PwDs). It replaced the earlier Persons with Disabilities (Equal Opportunities, Protection of Rights, and Full Participation) Act, 1995; aligning Indian laws with the UNCRPD, to which India is a signatory. The Act stresses on equality and nondiscrimination of persons with disabilities.

The section on healthcare (Chapter V.25) highlights the following:

> *The appropriate Government and the local authorities shall take necessary measures for the persons with disabilities to provide: (a) free healthcare in the vicinity, especially in rural area subject to such family income as may be notified; (b) barrier-free access in all parts of Government and*

private hospitals and other healthcare institutions and centers; (c) priority in attendance and treatment.

CURRENT SCENARIO

Even though there are many Laws and Acts to protect the rights of people with disabilities and initiatives to provide them equal opportunities, it is sad to note that they are not fully understood and made use of by those concerned. The medical fraternity to whom persons with disabilities turn up to is understandably not well versed with the various provisions provided in the Acts, to offer guidance to the people.

Until about 20 years back, cardiac surgeries were deferred in children with DS despite governments promoting inclusion in healthcare. This was mainly because of the resource limited, crowded healthcare setup in developing countries where there is a long waiting list for cardiac and other surgeries, leading to triaging and prioritization. But in the current era, children with DS are not sidelined or surgeries postponed just because of the presence of the extra chromosome.

Still, it may be seen that at times treatment is withheld or postponed because the treatment and the outcome are futile. This is not only seen in DS but in other conditions also. The term "futility" has been frequently discussed in medical and ethics literature over >30 years and has been generally dismissed as impossible to define; the term has been applied to so wide a variety of clinical situations that it is virtually incoherent. Nevertheless, it is still used in some situations to justify withholding curative or lifesaving treatments. Futility has many definitions, most of which are based on an individual's perception—"Clinically nonbeneficial" or "Medically inappropriate".

It is futile when a surgical procedure technically cannot be performed, or will not produce the desired physiologic effect, or it is highly unlikely to be efficacious, or is completely speculative and untried. Regardless of the presence or absence of DS, physicians must justify the care offered to patients by objectively assessing potential outcomes to avoid wasting resources on futile procedures. The concept of "killing" and "letting die" comes in here. Killing requires an action while letting die involves inaction. Letting the patient die is acceptable in medicine only under one of two conditions: the technology or surgical procedure is futile or the parents validly refuse the procedure. If neither of these conditions is satisfied letting the person die could be viewed morally as culpable negligence.

The day-to-day decision-making process in almost all circumstances remains in the domain of the family and caretakers, with the normative practice to follow the "best interests" standard. The inclusion of "in the treating physician's (or physicians') reasonable medical judgment" accommodates the normative practice.

SOLUTION

The way ahead is to take a decision that will better balance the legitimate interests of the child, the parents, the medical community, and society. An *Institutional Ethics Committee (IEC)* which most hospitals do have can be of help in taking difficult decisions or a *Hospital Medical Board* can be formed with representatives from the management, medical specialists, and experts from allied specialties. The IEC or the Medical Board should first verify that the best information available is being used. It should confirm the propriety of a decision that providers and parents have reached or confirm that the range of discretion accorded to the parents is appropriate. Then it should resolve disputes among those involved in a decision, by improving communication and understanding among them. Finally, when law and practice conflicts, actions in the courts usually provide guidance.

BASIC AWARENESS REQUIRED

The medical practitioner dealing with persons with disabilities should be aware of the various Acts, at least to some extent so that their patients can avail the benefits provided. The importance of a Unique Disability ID (UDID) card and the establishment of legal guardianship should be informed to the parents. So also, about the health insurance available to children with disabilities.

UDID card: It is provided by the government of India which gives them access to government benefits and schemes; but many are not aware of this and do not have the card.

Legal guardianship: It is a legal mechanism that allows for an individual to serve in a trusted role to make decisions for an adult with disabilities, to make personal and financial decisions on their behalf, and to serve the best interests of the disabled adult. Parents are the guardians for any child; but it ceases after the child becomes an adult at the age of 18 years. It is then mandatory that their parent (or parents) must apply for legal guardianship to be able to make decisions on behalf of their adult child with intellectual disabilities.

Niramaya Health Insurance Scheme: The scheme, as noted earlier provides affordable Health Insurance to PwDs with a cover of up to INR 1 lakh. There is facility for outpatient (OP) treatment from any hospital across the country, regular medical checkup for nonailing disabled, as well as ongoing therapies to reduce the impact of disability-related complications. This again is also not properly utilized mainly because of lack of awareness.

CONCLUSION

There are many Laws and Acts to protect the rights of persons with disabilities. But many of the caretakers and health care providers are not fully aware of the various aspects of it. The benefits of a UDID card and the mandate to get the legal guardianship registered in India should be advised to the caretakers by the health care providers. The Niramaya Health Insurance Scheme which covers even OP expenses is not availed by many, basically due to lack of awareness. It is the responsibility of all concerned to counsel the caretakers about the legal aspects and the benefits available for persons with disabilities.

Children with DS are born to humans; have the right to live with dignity and get the needed treatment as any other human—the fundamental right!

SUGGESTED READING

1. Disability Rights California. (2018). Sandra Jensen needed a heart-lung transplant, but several hospitals did not believe a woman with Down syndrome was a good candidate for surgery. [online] Available from https://www.disabilityrightsca.org/stories/sandra-jensen-needed-a-heart-lung-transplant-but-several-hospitals-did-not-believe-a-woman [Last accessed April, 2025].
2. Department of Empowerment of Persons with Disabilities. National Trust (Rules and Regulation). [online] Available from https://depwd.gov.in/document-category/national-trust-rules-regulation/ [Last accessed April, 2025].
3. Pless JE. The story of Baby Doe. N Engl J Med. 1983; 309(11):664.
4. The Rights of Persons with Disabilities Act, 2016. [online] Available from https://www.indiacode.nic.in/bitstream/123456789/15939/1/the_rights_of_persons_with_disabilities_act%2C_2016.pdf [Last accessed April, 2025].
5. The Persons with Disabilities Act, 1995. (1996). [online] Available from https://www.indiacode.nic.in/bitstream/123456789/8866/1/ind51207_%282%29disableact1995.pdf [Last accessed April, 2025].
6. United Nations, Department of Economic and Social Affairs. Convention on the Rights of Persons with Disabilities (CRPD). [online] Available from https://social.desa.un.org/issues/disability/crpd/convention-on-the-rights-of-persons-with-disabilities-crpd [Last accessed April, 2025].

CHAPTER 27

The Road Ahead

Shaji Thomas John

INTRODUCTION

The prevention and management of children with Down syndrome (DS) is a major research subject and numerous trials and research studies are being conducted worldwide to explore the various possibilities. These studies represent significant strides in understanding and developing treatments for DS. While some are in early research stages, others have progressed to clinical trials, offering hope for improved therapies in the future.

GENE THERAPY AND GENETIC INTERVENTIONS

With advances in genetics, there have been discussions about the potential use of gene editing to "correct" the chromosomal abnormality in DS. The potential gene editing approaches are:

- *Chromosome silencing (turning off the extra chromosome 21):* Researchers have experimented with inactivating the extra chromosome by inserting the *XIST* gene (X-inactive-specific transcript gene), which naturally silences one of the X chromosomes in females. In a 2013 study, scientists successfully silenced the extra chromosome 21 in laboratory cell cultures, opening the possibility of future treatments.
- *Epigenetic modifications (regulating gene expression):* Instead of removing the extra chromosome, some researchers aim to turn off or modify the expression of certain genes on chromosome 21. This could help reduce the severity of DS-related features without altering the entire genetic makeup.
- *CRISPR-Cas9 for targeted gene editing:* CRISPR-Cas9 (clustered regularly interspaced short palindromic repeats with CRISPR-associated protein 9) is a tool that allows precise editing of genes especially for single gene mutation. However, since trisomy 21 involves an entire extra chromosome, rather than a single faulty gene, CRISPR's traditional approach is challenging. Scientists are exploring ways to selectively modify specific genes on chromosome 21 that contribute to cognitive impairment, such as the *DYRK1A* gene, which is linked to brain development.

Considerable progress has been made in recent years, the most recent being that by Japanese researchers who utilized the *CRISPR-Cas9* gene-editing system to eliminate the extra chromosome 21 in test-tube-grown cells. The technique can identify which chromosome has been duplicated, so that it does not end up eliminating the wrong one and leaving the cell with two identical chromosomes. Instead, it leaves one from each parent. While promising in test tube experiments, the approach is not yet ready for testing in animals, in part because it can also leave changes in the retained chromosomes. Gene editing could cause off-target effects, leading to unintended consequences. Modifying genes in developed individuals (postnatal therapy) may have limited effectiveness compared to early intervention in embryos or fetuses. However, these successes have generated expectations that "gene editing" may someday ameliorate or eliminate many genetic conditions.

Ethical and Social Concerns

These rapid scientific advances have been accompanied by many ethical and social concerns about their implications. If gene editing is done in embryos, the changes could be passed on to future generations, raising ethical and societal concerns. National and international professional and ethics bodies have issued statements calling for additional basic research before genetic modification technologies are translated into clinical applications in humans, and highlighting the need to hear from stakeholders in these technologies. In particular, the needs and priorities of communities with firsthand experience of potentially targeted conditions are a critical consideration in clinical translation. Some argue that DS is a part of human diversity and that efforts should focus on supportive care rather than elimination of the condition.

ALZHEIMER DISEASE AND DOWN SYNDROME

Numerous studies have shown that by the age of 40 virtually 100% of people with DS will have the plaques and neurofibrillary tangles in the brain associated with Alzheimer disease (AD) but not necessarily the actual symptomatic disease. One study from 1989 indicated that 20–55% of people with DS will develop symptomatic AD before the age of 50. It was also noted later that 2–5% of people with DS developed dementia by the age of 40. But now there is evidence to show that people in their 30s or 40s do not develop dementia just because they have DS. The change in values reported have been attributed to diagnostic imprecision and overshadowing. Moreover, not all people with DS develop AD. Statistically, between 50 and 70% of people with DS will develop symptomatic AD by the age of 60. The exact proportion of people with DS who will develop Alzheimer's symptoms can vary based on genetic, environmental, and lifestyle factors, but the risk remains significantly higher than in the general population.

Given the high risk, individuals with DS should be monitored for signs of cognitive decline starting in their 30s. There are currently no specific treatments to prevent Alzheimer's in people with DS, but early intervention with supportive therapies can help manage symptoms and improve quality of life.

Various trials are being done with drugs that prevent Alzheimer disease-related plaque accumulation and improve cognitive function in individuals with DS. Donanemab is one such antiamyloid drug being studied in individuals with DS.

STUDIES TO IMPROVE COGNITION

Various drugs and megavitamin therapy with trace elements and antioxidants have been tried for cognitive improvement in DS. Recent research indicates that gonadotropin-releasing hormone (GnRH) therapies could improve cognitive functions by boosting brain connectivity in individuals with DS. Another study states that lipid nanoparticles can carry mRNA instructions into brain cells. Tiny particles of fat that can sneak protein-building instructions past the brain's blood-filtering system may someday enable new treatments. More work is needed to assess long-term safety and efficacy before these approaches can be tested in humans for treating AD, and other such conditions. Still, the findings "highlight the potential of lipid nanoparticles in overcoming one of the major challenges in treating brain diseases," which is to get past the blood-brain barrier.

FERTILITY AND CONCEPTION IN DOWN SYNDROME

The fertility status of individuals with DS varies between males and females, and is influenced by the genetic and physical characteristics associated with the condition. Women with DS are generally fertile and have the potential to conceive. However, fertility may be somewhat reduced compared to women without DS due to various factors, including hormonal imbalances and the presence of associated health issues.

Pregnancy in women with DS carries a higher risk of complications, such as miscarriage, preterm birth, and the birth of a child with DS or other chromosomal abnormalities. If a person with DS has a child, there is a 50% chance that the child will inherit an extracopy of chromosome 21. However, some pregnancies may result in miscarriage due to chromosomal abnormalities. Thus, there is a 35–50% chance that a child born to a mother with DS will also have DS. This percentage can vary depending on various factors, including the specific genetic mechanisms involved in the parent's DS (e.g., whether it is a full trisomy 21, mosaicism, or a translocation). While the most significant risk is for DS, there is also a slightly increased risk of other chromosomal abnormalities or genetic conditions in the offspring, although this is less well-documented. These could include conditions that result from other chromosomal aneuploidies (e.g., trisomy 13 or trisomy 18), although such occurrences are relatively rare compared to DS.

Some children born to parents with DS (about 50%) will have a typical chromosome count (46 chromosomes without the extra chromosome 21). However, these children may still require monitoring for health issues as they may have a higher risk of developmental issues due to genetic, environmental, or prenatal factors. The incidence of such outcomes is not well-quantified as there is limited statistical data available on these issues due to the rarity of pregnancies involving parents with DS. Most information comes from case studies and small research groups, so the exact percentages can vary depending on the population studied.

Most males with DS have significantly reduced fertility or are infertile. Although extremely rare, there have been a few documented cases of men with DS fathering children. However, this is an exception rather than the norm. In the rare cases where this occurs, theoretically the child could either have DS, another chromosomal abnormality, or be chromosomally typical. The reduced fertility is primarily due to partial gonadal dysfunction with issues such as low sperm count, poor sperm motility, and other anatomical or hormonal factors. Men with DS appear to experience a normal puberty, which starts at the usual age. After puberty, however, the testicular volume falls, the production of gonadotropins rises, and the gonadal dysfunction worsens with age. The increased production of luteinizing hormones and follicle-stimulating hormones and decreased production of anti-Müllerian hormone evidence the Sertoli and Leydig cell dysfunction.

Social Considerations

The reproductive choices of individuals with DS should be respected, and they should have access to the same reproductive rights and medical care as the general population. More and more individuals with DS are getting married around the world and the question of having an offspring is usually brought up to the physician. Genetic counseling is highly recommended for families under these circumstances where a prospective parent with DS is involved. The risks and outcomes should be fully explained to them. Individuals with DS who are of reproductive age should be provided with comprehensive support, including education about sexuality, reproductive health, and the potential challenges of parenthood.

SUPPORT GROUPS

Support groups play a crucial role in the lives of individuals with many diseases, their families, and caregivers. These groups provide emotional, informational, social, and advocacy support, helping families navigate challenges, and celebrate milestones.

Providing emotional support is one of the greatest benefits of a support group. Support groups offer a sense of belonging and reassurance that others share similar experiences and reduces the feeling of isolation in the parents. Hearing success stories and experiences from others can be inspiring and uplifting; and provides hope and encouragement. It also provides a platform for learning about the latest updates in the management of children with DS. Experts can guide the parents and children about educational aspects and the prospects of taking up a vocation as the child grows. Issues related to legal aspects and the current laws and their importance, especially government benefits and disability rights, can be discussed in the group which will be of immense benefit to the parents and caretakers.

Since persons with DS are not able to form a group to voice their needs, the support groups can act on their behalf and advocate for policy changes and fight for their rights. They can also educate the society about the nature of DS and help to break down stereotypes in the community. The groups can provide opportunities for participation and conduct awareness campaigns to promote inclusion in society.

Every pediatrician/healthcare provider comes in contact with a large number of children/persons with DS and a support group should be formed in every district and have regular meetings. The Indian Academy of Pediatrics (IAP) has decided to form a DS support group in every town where there is an IAP branch. A president and secretary can be elected from the parents and the group can meet at regular intervals with the support of the IAP branch. Regular sessions by doctors, therapists, educators, and involvement of public figures and legal experts can go a long way in fulfilling the needs of the group. Few of the parents can be trained to be counselors and they may be contacted to offer support to mothers who have newly diagnosed babies with DS.

TRANSITION OF CARE

Transition of care (ToC) is defined as "a purposeful, planned, process that addresses the medical, psychosocial, educational, and vocational needs of adolescents and young adults especially with chronic medical conditions as they advance from a pediatric and family centered to an adult individual focused healthcare provider".

The ToC leads to better satisfaction and leads to improved treatment adherence and improved selfcare. Doctor should address medical, psychosocial, educational, and vocational needs.

Most children with DS and other similar conditions do not receive the support they need in the transition. Children with medical and developmental issues have an increased susceptibility to emerging or worsening of chronic health conditions, which should be understood by the health personnel who takes over the child.

Barriers to Transition of Care

The main barrier is the difficulty in leaving their pediatric clinician and therapist; as there is a long-standing relationship that makes it difficult to totally cut off from them. There is also a lack of adult clinicians with interest to care for youth with pediatric-onset conditions. Moreover, there is an anxiety on the part of the care-giver about communication, coordination, practice styles, and changing therapies.

The transition policy must be discussed with the parents/caregivers right from mid-adolescent age and it should be a gradual process. It is the duty of the pediatrician to teach the child the basic life skills such as communication skills, functional mathematics, and functional reading so that they can be on their own in later life. Identifying emotions and social skills are important to help them live in an inclusive society. Vocational training and career planning should be given with anticipatory guidance and parenting support. A detailed summary should be prepared and handed over to the adult physician and gradually integrated to adult care. Feedback should be elicited both from the physician and the child and progress should be monitored for some time to give the family the confidence that they will be properly taken care of in the years to come.

Assisted Living

Equipment and facilities for assisted living are required when people with disabilities need support to enhance independence and improve quality of life. They may need—(1) assisted living devices when complications of the various systemic problems surface as age advances and (2) assisted living facilities (ALFs).

- *The assisted living devices include:*
  - Mobility aids such as wheelchairs, walkers, canes, and orthotics
  - Communication aids such as hearing aids, screen readers, and speech generating devices (SGDs)
  - Sensory aids such as magnifiers, large print books and materials, and alerting devices
  - Other assistive devices such as adaptive utensils, adaptive writing tools, cognitive aids (manage memory, attention, etc.), eye-tracking devices (control computers using eye movements), personal assistants (Google home, Alexa, HomePod, etc.)
- *ALF:* One of the common questions asked by parents and caretakers is related to the future status of these children/persons with DS when the caretakers are no longer there to support and care for them. This is where ALFs have a role to play. These are residential facilities where older children and adults with DS may live when they are unable to live safely or comfortably in a home of their own. There are even living facilities where they can move in with their parents, to a community living atmosphere where they do have other families with similar issues. They can stay on after the demise of their parents and they do not have to relocate to another home thereby preventing the added trauma of adjustment to a new environment.

They live in their own rooms or apartments and share common areas. They get help with activities of daily living and have services that typically include meals, housekeeping, medication, and social activities. There is safety and supervision in a secure environment and there is social and community engagement. They permit residents to age in place and is an example of a "social model" of care.

CONCLUSION

Numerous trials and researches are conducted worldwide to correct the abnormality or alleviate the symptoms associated with DS. Chromosomal silencing, epigenetic modifications, and CRISPR-Cas9 for targeted gene editing are some of the promising ones being studied, but they are still in the trial phases. Ethical and social concerns have also to be addressed in these researches. Fertility and conception are also matters of importance as more and more persons with DS are getting married in the present age. Support groups are of immense benefit to parents/caretakers, and groups may be formed, if not available, with the help of academic and voluntary organizations. And finally, it is the duty of all doctors to facilitate a proper transition of care as the child grows up to an adult.

SUGGESTED READING

1. Grinspon RP, Bedecarrás P, Ballerini MG, Iñiguez G, Rocha A, Mantovani Rodrigues Resende EA, et al. Early onset of primary hypogonadism revealed by serum anti-Mullerian hormone determination during infancy and childhood in trisomy 21. Int J Androl. 2011;34:e487-98.

2. Haveman M, Maaskant MA, van Schrojenstein Lantman-de Valk HMJ. Epidemiological aspects of mental handicap in children in a region of the Netherlands. Australia New Zealand J Develop Disabil. 1989;15(3): 241-55.
3. Michie M, Allyse M. Gene modification therapies: views of parents of people with Down syndrome. Genet Med. 2019;21:487-92.
4. Parizot E, Dard R, Janel N, Vialard F. Down syndrome and infertility: what support should we provide? J Assist Reprod Genet. 2019;36(6):1063-7.
5. van den Driessen Mareeuw FA, Coppus AMW, Delnoij DMJ, de Vries E. Quality of health care according to people with Down syndrome, their parents and support staff-A qualitative exploration. J Appl Res Intellect Disabil. 2020;33(3):496-514.
6. Zigman WB, Devenny DA, Krinsky-McHale SJ, Jenkins EC, Urv TK, Wegiel J. Alzheimer's Disease in Adults with Down Syndrome. Int Rev Res Ment Retard. 2008;36:103-45.
7. Zimmerman S, Carder P, Schwartz L, Silbersack J, Temkin-Greener H, Thomas KS. The Imperative to Reimagine Assisted Living. J Am Med Dir Assoc. 2022;23(2):225-34.

CHAPTER 28

Success Stories

Shaji Thomas John

INTRODUCTION

The success stories of individuals with Down syndrome (DS) are shared to highlight the fact that, with proper nurturing, children and adults with DS can lead fulfilling lives and participate meaningfully in an inclusive society. Many have gone on to achieve significant milestones as young adults. Identifying their interests and talents, combined with strong parental support and timely guidance from healthcare professionals, can make all the difference. One memorable example is the 2019 film "The Peanut Butter Falcon," in which Zack Gottsagen, an actor with DS, played the lead role. The following are a few such inspiring stories that illustrate their achievements and the dedication that helped them thrive.

DHANYA VIJAYAN

Dhanya grew up as a student of a local normal government school much before we started advocating that these children should be sent to normal schools. She was fascinated with the classical dance form "Bharatanatyam" which she used to witness during the school programs. She told her father her wish and the father sought professional dance teachers to coach her. It was difficult to get a dance teacher initially to train a child with DS, but one renowned teacher agreed to try and teach her Bharatanatyam. Her father used to go with her to the dance classes and memorize the steps the teacher taught the students. He used to come home and make her rehearse the steps. It was a tough job; and to add to that, some of the parents of other students ridiculed him for trying to teach a clumsy student like her and waste their time also. But that only made him more determined; and her daughter thoroughly enjoyed the dance classes. As the months passed on, she became an expert dancer and she won her school Bharatanatyam competition during the youth festival for 3 years in a row competing with other typically developed children. She is now a dance teacher in a school and doing extremely well. All credits to her love for the dance and the determined nature of her father **(Figs. 1A and B)**.

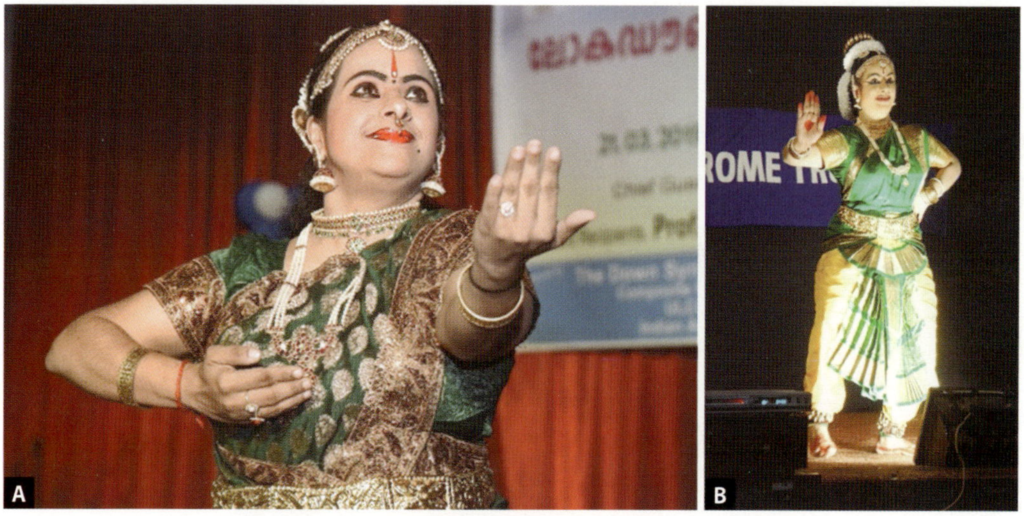

Figs. 1A and B: (A) Dance by Dhanya Vijayan; (B) Bharatanatyam by Dhanya Vijayan.

ANITA RAMDAS

Anita was brought to me at the age of 3 months with respiratory infection. She had a congenital heart disease and by that time, her mother had taken her to very many doctors in various places. She was disappointed that the doctors did not give a positive projection about the future of the child. It was in the 1990s and therapy centers were limited. Her mother wanted to do the best for her and her father took up a job in Dubai to give a better education and training for her. As she grew up, they found that Anita had a passion for modeling. They encouraged her and her institution supported her. She was trained to be a model and soon she became a model and calendar girl in Dubai. They returned a few years later and she has modeled for textile mills and tabletop calendars in India **(Figs. 2A to F)**.

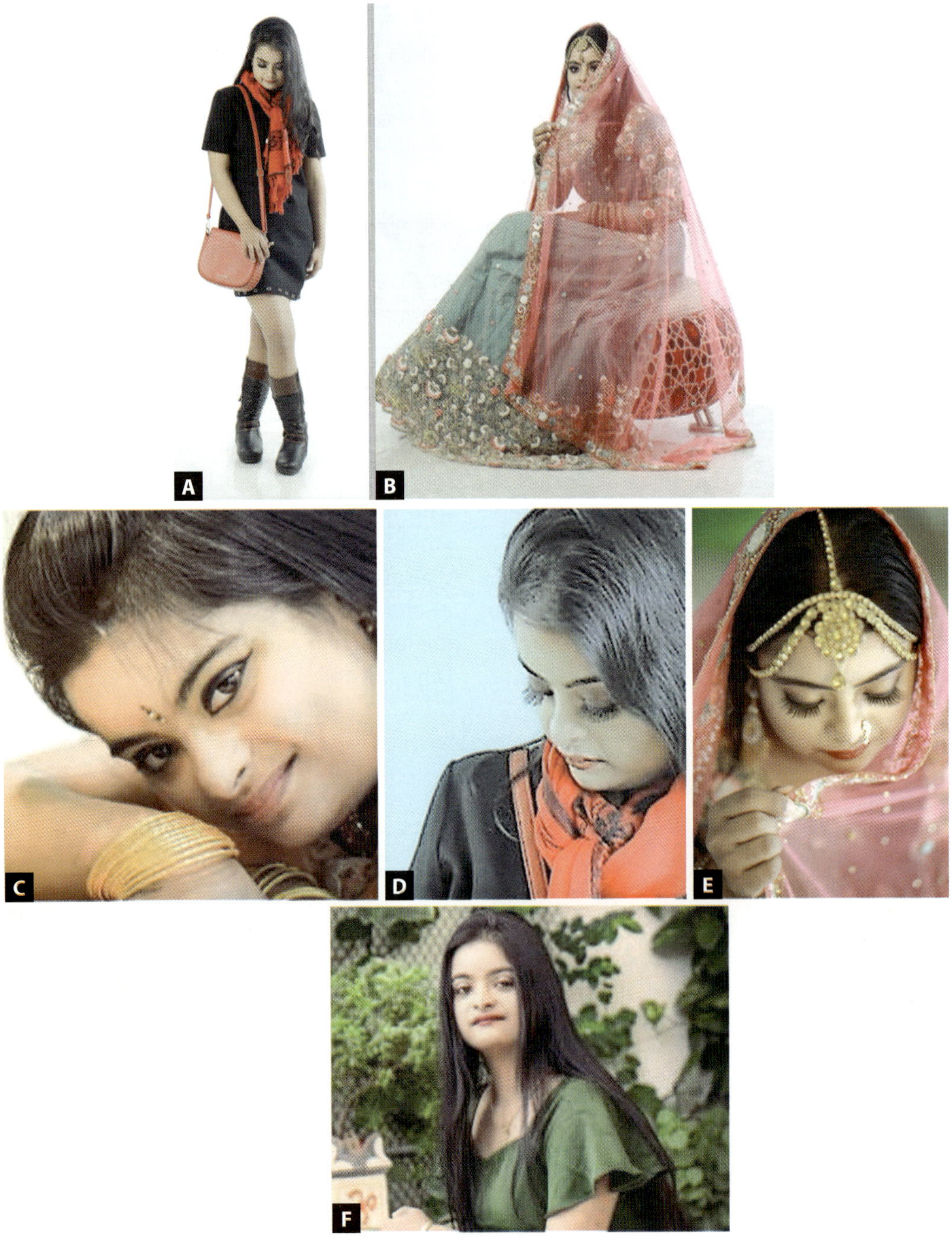

Figs. 2A to F: Anita Ramdas as a model.

GOPIKRISHNAN K VARMA

Gopi was a very energetic boy when I first met him in early 2000. His father got a transfer to provide the needed support for his son. He had tremendous stamina and like most children with DS, a passion for music and dancing. He liked imitating people and acting, and did a lot of reels with the help of his mother. He loved seeing movies but was more interested in the making of a film after seeing any movie. Gopi later got a chance to play the lead role in the movie "Thirike" along with two other persons with DS. He became a celebrity after that and has by now acted in four movies, the latest being the Bollywood movie "Sitaare Zameen Par". His mother is the driving force behind him who trains him before every shoot of the movie **(Figs. 3A to C)**.

OTHER STARS

There are many others from all over the country: like Ismail whose fascination for magic made him a stage magician **(Fig. 4)**, Ameen who worked as a florist in a shop in the Middle East later came back to India and became the loving tea vendor whose customers went to him just to see his smile **(Fig. 5)**, and Alan who graduated in Hotel Management is now working in a star hotel in the Middle East **(Fig. 6)**. We also have a Handicrafts emporium run exclusively by women with DS **(Figs. 7 and 8)**.

We also have sports enthusiast like Naghash **(Figs. 9 and 10)** who is working in a confectionary production line and Yoga experts like Ann Mooken **(Fig. 11)** who has been recognized by the state government. Many of them are medalists in the Down syndrome National Games

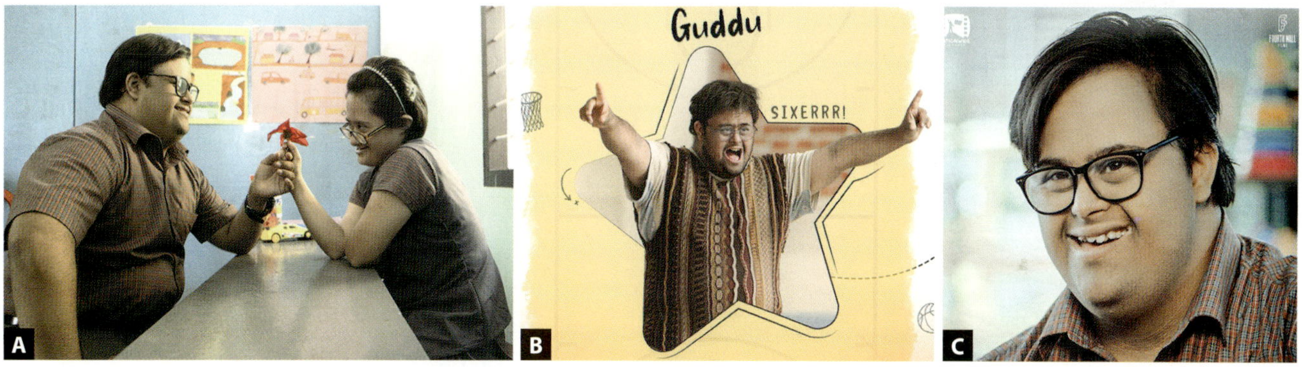

Figs. 3A to C: Gopikrishnan in various movies.

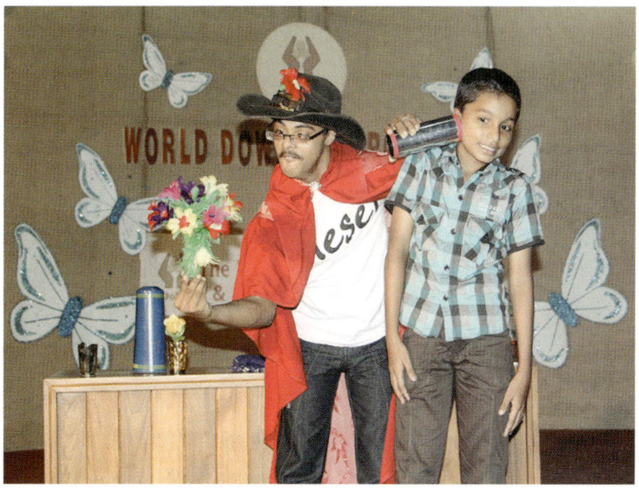

Fig. 4: Ismail the stage magician.

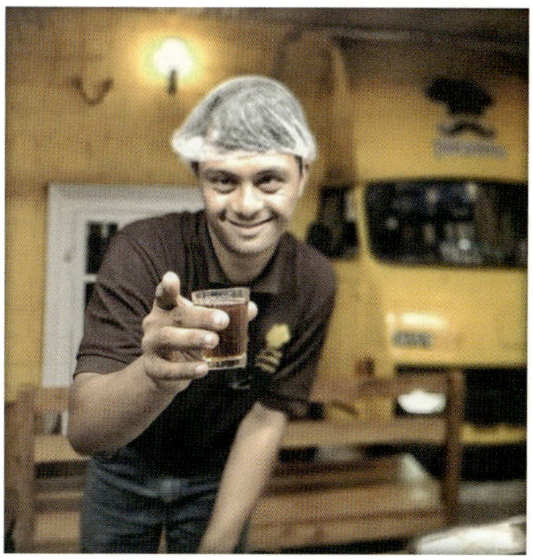

Fig. 5: Ameen in his teashop.

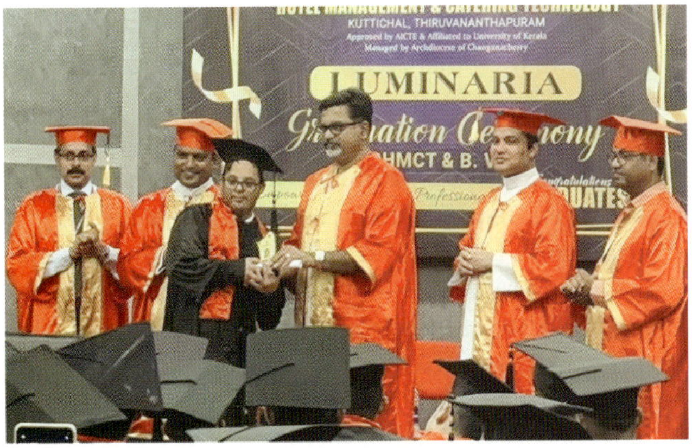

Fig. 6: Alan on his graduation.

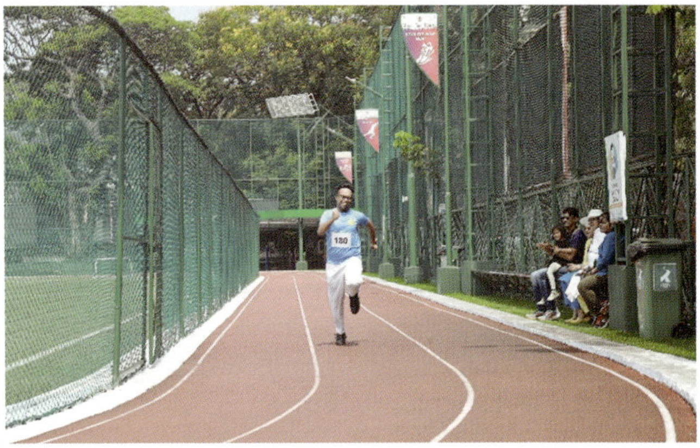

Fig. 9: Naghash on the tracks.

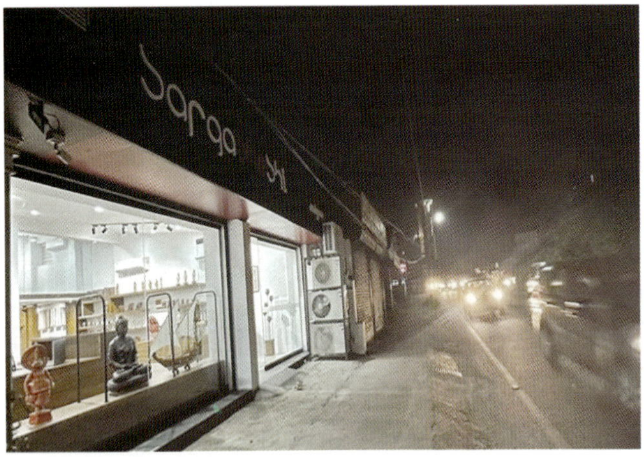

Fig. 7: Sargasheshi: The handicrafts emporium managed exclusively by women with DS.

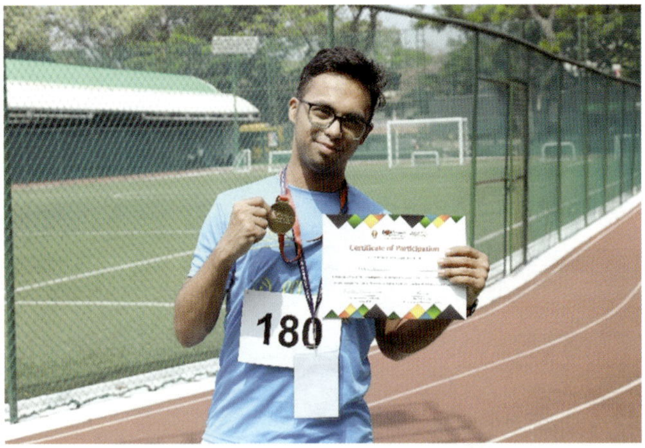

Fig. 10: Naghash exhibiting his medals.

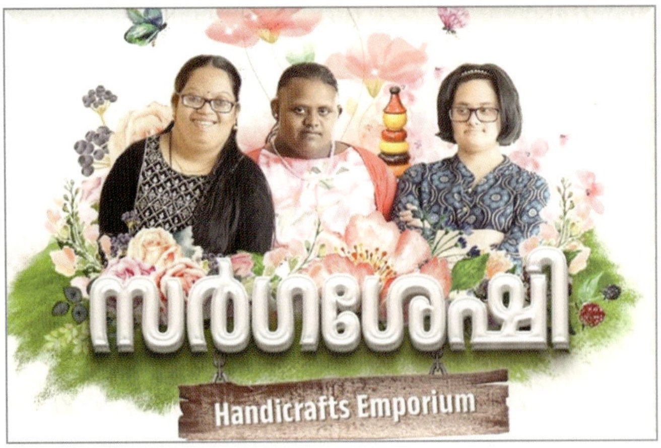

Fig. 8: The women who manage the emporium—Sargasheshi.

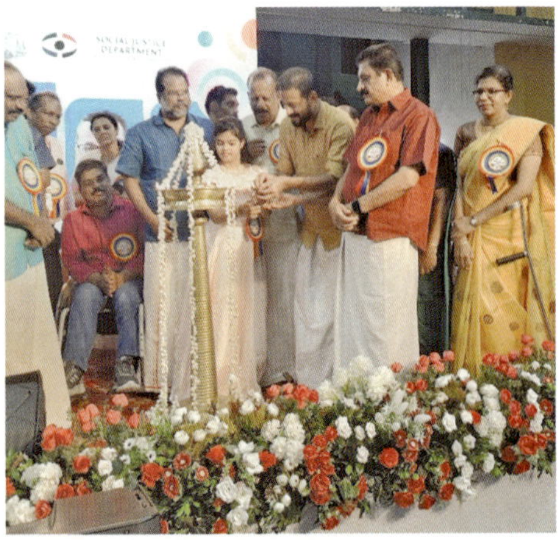

Fig. 11: Ann recognized by the government.

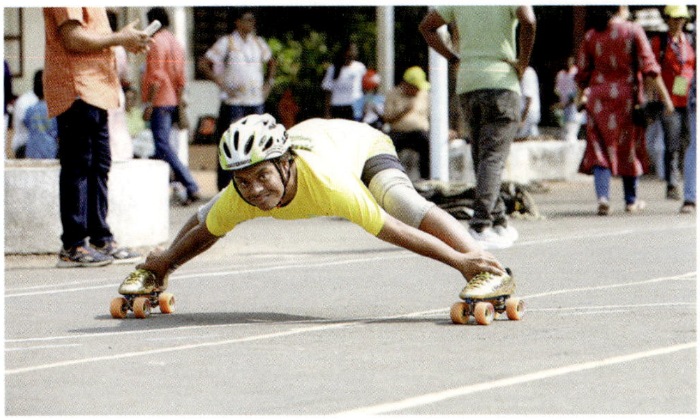

Fig. 12: Sanju: Roller Skating winner at the DS National Games 2025.

organized yearly by the Down Syndrome Federation of India **(Fig. 12)** and the Special Olympics for persons with Intellectual Disabilities organized by Special Olympics—Bharat **(Fig. 13)**.

Notable individuals with DS who have made it in the international arena include: K. Rishitha (Silver Medal in Roller Skating at International Special Olympics in Berlin, 2023); Sneha Verma (Gold Medal in Powerlifting at the Special Olympics in Los Angels, 2015); and Priyanka Dewan (Gold Medal in Roller Skating at the Special Olympics in Abu Dhabi, 2019).

There are many more in the list and they all have one thing in common: they have an extra 21st chromosome and a supportive family and teachers who believed in them. An early and sustained interventional program with proper medical care can do wonders for these children and help them live a fulfilling life.

The World Down Syndrome Day observed every year on March 21st helps to promote and showcase the talents of persons with DS and break the stereotype image in the minds of the public.

CONCLUSION

Many individuals with DS are leading fulfilling lives, having pursued their dreams with the unwavering

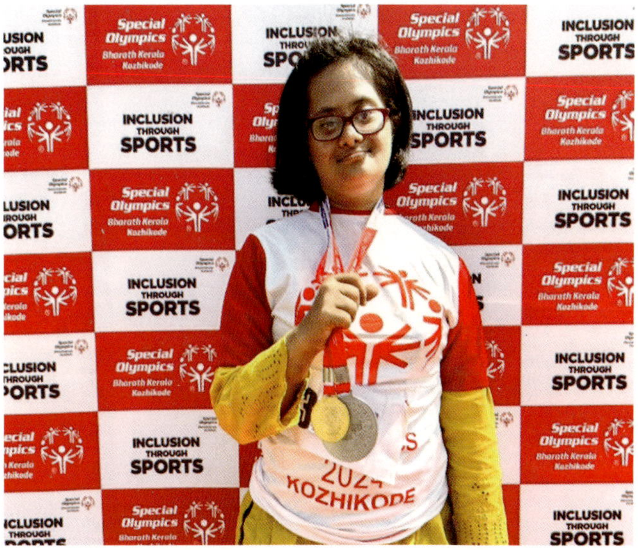

Fig. 13: Tina at the Special Olympics with her medals.

support of their parents, well-wishers, and healthcare professionals. Several are engaged in meaningful employment and contributing actively to society. What is essential is creating awareness among caregivers and the broader community to foster an environment where persons with DS can live inclusive, empowered lives.

SUGGESTED READING

Since these are personal stories, only few media news are available

1. https://www.thenewsminute.com/kerala/gopikrishnan-sets-record-first-down-syndrome-actor-play-lead-thirike-150188
2. https://www.onmanorama.com/lifestyle/women/2018/12/13/anitha-a--special-child-with-a-story.html
3. https://newzhook.com/story/dhanya-vijayan-down-syndrome -kerala-disabled/
4. https://www.newindianexpress.com/good-news/2022/Sep/25/down-with-down-syndrome-but-nothing-stops-this-keralabharatanatyam-dancer-2501594.html
5. https://30stades.com/society/kerala-sargasheshi-handicraft-breaks-stereotypes-employs-women-with-down-syndrome-inclusive-2407776

Epilogue

Down syndrome (DS) is a genetic condition for which there is currently no definitive cure, although extensive research is ongoing globally. Clinical presentations can be atypical, and co-existing medical conditions are common, often resulting in diagnostic overshadowing. The increased prevalence of associated health issues in individuals with DS necessitates a high index of clinical suspicion and a comprehensive approach to evaluation. Early diagnosis and prompt intervention remain the cornerstones of effective management. Regular follow-up is essential, and the implementation of structured care charts, such as the one presented in **Table 1**, can be particularly valuable. As children with DS transition into adolescence and adulthood, ensuring continuity of care becomes increasingly important. Assisted living options may offer substantial support for older individuals. Parents should be counseled about the prevailing laws and other legal aspects that support them. With timely medical care, tailored therapies, and adequate social support, many individuals with DS can grow into responsible adults who lead independent and meaningful lives.

TABLE 1: Follow-up of important medical issues in children with Down syndrome till 18 years of age.

	At birth	*6 months*	*1 year*	*2 years*	*3 years*	*4 years*	*5 years*	*6–9 years*	*10–18 years*
Karyotyping and genetic counseling	✓	–	–	–	–	–	–	–	–
Echocardiography	✓	–	–	–	–	–	–	–	–
Thyroid function tests	✓	✓	✓	✓	✓	✓	✓	✓[a]	✓[a]
CBC and PBS	✓	–	✓	✓	✓	✓	✓	–	–
Audiology/hearing	✓	✓	–	✓[c]	✓	✓	✓	✓[b]	✓[b]
Ophthalmology	✓	–	–	✓	–	✓	–	✓[b]	✓[b]
Dental	–	–	✓	✓	✓	✓	✓	✓[a]	✓[a]
Testicular examination	–	–	–	✓	✓	✓	✓	✓[a]	✓[a]
Growth/development	✓	✓	✓	✓	✓	✓	✓	✓[a]	✓[a]

Notes: ✓ indicates evaluation to be done; – indicates evaluation not to be done, unless clinically indicated.

[a]Every year.

[b]Once in 2 years.

[c]At 2 years if not done at 18 months. Routine vaccinations should not be skipped; and the need for pneumococcal conjugate/polysaccharide vaccine, influenza and varicella vaccines should be stressed. Evaluation and investigations to be done more frequently, if warranted.

(CBC: complete blood count; PBS: peripheral blood smear)

Source: John ST, Gayathri K, Ahmed S, Multtani KS, Menon PSN, Kumar RK, et al. Consensus Statement of the Neurodevelopmental Pediatrics Chapter of Indian Academy of Pediatrics (IAP) on the Management of Children With Down Syndrome. Indian Pediatr. 2023;60(4):298-307.

Index

Page numbers followed by *f* refer to figure, *fc* refer to flowchart, and *t* refer to table.

L

M

N

O

P